Praise for *Percolate*

*"How can an aardvark and a platypus help you change your life? How can #WWBWD help you make better decisions? And what does brewing coffee have to do with being healthier and happier? For the answers to these and other life-altering questions, look no further than **Percolate**, Elizabeth Hamilton-Guarino's masterwork. I highly recommend this book if you want to live more fully, laugh more heartily, and leave a lasting legacy for your loved ones!"*

— **Noah St. John,** best-selling author of *The Book of AFFORMATIONS®*, www.NoahStJohn.com

"For years I have enjoyed bringing clarity and joy into my life by taking time each morning to reflect on my blessings over a hot cup of coffee. Now I have a new favorite way to 'percolate,' thanks to this wonderful book! After following Elizabeth on The Best Ever Your Network, I am so happy that she has found a new way to share her inspirational message with us all!"

— **Michelle Phillips,** best-selling author of *The Beauty Blueprint*, www.MichellePhillips.com

"Elizabeth shows us how to follow our heart, show up for ourselves, and have the courage to really be ourselves—that we've been percolating all along."

— **Gary Kobat,** international authority on integrative well-being

*"What amazing miracles have been percolating in your life that you might not realize, expect, or understand? Elizabeth and Katie will help you find out in **Percolate**. Enjoy the experience of letting your best self filter through!"*

— **Deb Scott,** host of *The Best People We Know Radio Show*

"I love the Java Jive, and it loves me . . . and I really love **Percolate**, a bold and flavorful blend of higher wisdom, experience, and common sense. Drink deep of this rich brew, and you'll enjoy life to the fullest."

— **Stephen Powers,** Grammy Award–winning producer and co-founder of Agape Media International

"**Percolate** is a gift—a marvelous one— filled with intelligence and beauty."

— **Michael McGlone,** actor

"Courageously awaken and percolate your best self forward, and remember to put a fresh filter of unconditional love and light in each day."

— **Debra Oakland,** author and founder of Living in Courage

"If you can't wait to get your hands on another self-help book filled with dogma and strict directions, then **Percolate** isn't for you. However, if you've been searching for a book that can brilliantly guide you to guide yourself, search no more."

— **Gabe Berman,** author of Live Like a Fruit Fly

"**Percolate** is not another self-help book. It's an invitation to sit down with Elizabeth Hamilton-Guarino for a cup of java and a generous helping of real-life stories that just may shift something in your own life—it's that powerful."

— **Lisa Tener,** award-winning book coach

"Put down this book if you don't want to do the work."

— **Fred Cuellar,** Diamond Cutters International

*"Just like the ingredients of an excellent cup of coffee, **Percolate** delivers the perfect blend of emotional energy, spiritual spice, and tremendously good taste. Elizabeth's bubbly attitude and fresh perspective will leave you thirsty for more!"*

— **Sue Jacques,** the Civility CEO®

*"It takes only moments to learn that Elizabeth Hamilton-Guarino has a gift for connecting with people. She shares her own personal experiences, and those of others, in a way that challenges each of us to become our best. The stories in **Percolate** continue to express her inspirational spirit and will simply make you feel good."*

— **Sarah C. Bazey,** Mrs. International 2012 and president and CEO of Simplex Construction Supplies, Inc.

*"**Percolate** is the perfect title for Elizabeth's book because anyone who knows her personality will agree that she is like a constant, contagious, and inspirational jolt of caffeine. This is a woman who lives every minute of every day to the fullest. Elizabeth's cup runneth over, and if we can sip in just a little bit of her wisdom and experience, we should consider ourselves lucky!"*

— **Anthony Turk,** Hollywood publicist

"Elizabeth's inspirational and caring spirit is reflected on each and every page of this book. A special thank-you to Elizabeth for guiding us on this journey to our best selves."

— **Lisa Cocuzza,** founder of It's a Glam Thing

"Are you happy? Are you living a life that you love? If not, Elizabeth Hamilton-Guarino is your new best friend, and it's time that you meet! In her own unique and delightful style, Elizabeth shows how to create your best-ever life, no matter what your personal circumstances."

— **Gina Clowes,** author of *One of the Gang: Nurturing the Souls of Children with Food Allergies,* www.AllergyMoms.com

PERCOLATE

Hay House Titles of Related Interest

YOU CAN HEAL YOUR LIFE, the movie,
starring Louise Hay & Friends
(available as a 1-DVD program and
an expanded 2-DVD set)
Watch the trailer at: www.LouiseHayMovie.com

THE SHIFT, the movie, **starring Dr. Wayne W. Dyer**
(available as a 1-DVD program and
an expanded 2-DVD set)
Watch the trailer at: www.DyerMovie.com

*THE BEAUTY BLUEPRINT: 8 Steps to Building the Life
and Look of Your Dreams,* by Michelle Phillips

*EXCUSES BEGONE! How to Change Lifelong, Self-Defeating
Thinking Habits,* by Dr. Wayne W. Dyer

SOUL COACHING®: 28 Days to Discover Your Authentic Self,
by Denise Linn

*TAPPING THE POWER WITHIN: A Path to Self-Empowerment
for Women,* by Iyanla Vanzant

WHAT IS YOUR SELF-WORTH? A Woman's Guide to Validation,
by Cheryl Saban

YOU CAN CREATE AN EXCEPTIONAL LIFE,
by Louise Hay and Cheryl Richardson

All of the above are available at your local bookstore, or may be
ordered by visiting: Hay House USA: www.hayhouse.com®; Hay
House Australia: www.hayhouse.com.au; Hay House UK: www
.hayhouse.co.uk; Hay House South Africa: www.hayhouse.co.za;
Hay House India: www.hayhouse.co.in

PERCOLATE

Let Your Best Self Filter Through

Elizabeth Hamilton-Guarino

Also Includes "Coffee Breaks"
with Dr. Katie Eastman

HAY HOUSE, INC.
Carlsbad, California • New York City
London • Sydney • Johannesburg
Vancouver • Hong Kong • New Delhi

Published and distributed in the United States by: Hay House, Inc.: www
.hayhouse.com® • *Published and distributed in Australia by:* Hay House Australia Pty. Ltd.: www.hayhouse.com.au • *Published and distributed in the
United Kingdom by:* Hay House UK, Ltd.: www.hayhouse.co.uk • *Published
and distributed in the Republic of South Africa by:* Hay House SA (Pty), Ltd.:
www.hayhouse.co.za • *Distributed in Canada by:* Raincoast Books: www
.raincoast.com • *Published in India by:* Hay House Publishers India: www
.hayhouse.co.in

Cover design: Sandra Waugh • *Interior design:* Tricia Breidenthal
Interior illustrations: Sandra Waugh

Library of Congress Cataloging-in-Publication Data

Hamilton-Guarino, Elizabeth, date.
 Percolate : let your best self filter through / Elizabeth Hamilton-Guarino, with
Dr. Katie Eastman. -- 1st edition.
 pages cm
 ISBN 978-1-4019-4298-4 (tradepaper : alk. paper) 1. Change (Psychology)
2. Self-actualization (Psychology) 3. Self-realization. I. Eastman, Katie, date.
II. Title.
 BF637.C4H34 2014
 158.1--dc23
                                        2013042355

Tradepaper ISBN: 978-1-4019-4298-4

17 16 15 14   4 3 2 1
1st edition, April 2014

SUSTAINABLE
FORESTRY
INITIATIVE

Certified Chain of Custody
Promoting Sustainable Forestry
www.sfiprogram.org
SFI-01268

SFI label applies to the text stock

Printed in the United States of America

To my husband, Peter, and our four boys
— Elizabeth

To John and Cali
— Dr. Katie

CONTENTS

Percolate (verb):
To filter gradually through
a porous surface or substance.
Spread gradually through
an area or group of people.

— OXFORD ENGLISH DICTIONARY

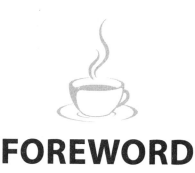

FOREWORD

Of all the self-empowerment books, from all the books, in all the stores, you've chosen this one. If that sounds familiar, it's my take on the infamous line by Humphrey Bogart's character, Rick, in *Casablanca*. And if you don't know that, or if you just said "Who's Humphrey Bogart?" then it's probably past your bedtime, you need to finish your homework, and you haven't lived long enough to need a book like *Percolate* just yet.

Life is challenging. The massive pool of self-help, inspirational, empowerment, and psychological studies books on the market is proof that people are searching for ways to cope, laugh, solve problems, and simply improve or change their world. Since you're reading this book, or considering whether it's worth your time to continue reading this book, you're one of those people. Good for you for being proactive and seeking out some sense of direction. Instead, you could just sit on your couch with a bottle of Jack and a can of honey-roasted peanuts while channel flipping and catching glimpses of before-and-after makeovers and sound bites from Dr. Oz that make you think to yourself, *At least I'm not that bad.* No? Just me?

In your quest for a good read, how do you decide on what to add to your real and virtual bookshelves? How big are your problems? What can *Percolate* offer you that no other book can? I can only help you answer one of those three questions, and yes, it's the last one. *Percolate* will bring you a relatable perspective, humor and personality, and words weighted with genuine inspiration to get results.

The author, Elizabeth Hamilton-Guarino, doesn't wear a stethoscope or sit in a chair and ask, "How does that make you feel?" She, along with terrific contributions from Dr. Katie Eastman, speaks as a mom, friend, daughter, sister, co-worker, and victim-turned-champion. Elizabeth is just like you and me, with ups and downs in life, and she's come through some rough times with lessons to share. But what separates her from us is that she took action by creating and establishing a phenomenal online network called Best Ever You so that she can help people discover their authentic selves and live their best lives.

Whether it's her radio show, magazine, or website postings, Elizabeth speaks from the heart and provides access to advice and opinions from people that you'd otherwise never meet. Now she brings us *Percolate,* a book about courage, pushing past fear, and never giving up. I'm in!

Admittedly, I'm not a famous person, and you likely have never heard of me. I did some research on the subject of writing a Foreword for a book, and it's advised that I give you some of my background info in hopes that it lends credibility to what I'm saying. So, here's a little bit about me:

I've been in the entertainment business for 20 years and am a talent manager/producer. The first eight years of my career were spent representing comedic talent (stand-ups, actors, writers) and, most notably, I discovered Jimmy Fallon and helped developed his career from before and through his *SNL* years. I was also fortunate to serve as the script supervisor on three of Adam Sandler's comedy albums, along with one of Pauly Shore's; my creative brain was taking me in new directions. When I decided to move on from managing other people's careers, I began to focus on my own, and in the last decade I've held the following positions: EVP Talent and Development and Executive Producer at National Lampoon; Head of Special Projects and Marketing Initiatives for Comic Relief 2006; Executive in Charge of Alternative Comedy Programming for The Fred Silverman Company; and Director of Comedy

Relations and Content at Myspace. I have now returned to management and am also a social-media consultant; seminar host for multiple entertainment subjects; and a script consultant for film, TV, stand-up, and sketch. In addition, I'm an adjunct professor at Boston University and teach a class in talent representation and contracts. In 2011, my class had the honor of being ranked sixth in The Daily Beast's Hottest College Courses in the Country.

I met Elizabeth when she interviewed my client Frank Stallone for her radio show. She interviewed me on her radio show also, and then Frank graced the cover of the December 2012 issue of *Best Ever You* magazine. Elizabeth was highly impressive as a hardworking, dedicated professional whose passion for her projects instantly garnered my respect.

That uncomfortable summation of my life leads me to this: I've probably read a couple thousand scripts, treatments, jokes, sketches, ideas, and books over the course of my career. It's difficult to find material that's both well written and sincere and engaging. *Percolate* is not only a great read, but Elizabeth also lays her heart at your feet, relates to you as an equal, and provides workbook-style tools for you to execute the advice she's giving. It rings true when she says "Nobody can force you to believe in yourself," and she makes the concept of change attainable so that you can take action in your own life without feeling lost, overwhelmed, or discouraged. Not many writers can accomplish that.

One of the things I like the most about Elizabeth's style is how direct she is. She's the mother of four boys, so it stands to reason that she's had to learn to cut to the chase in many conversations. Some of my favorite things she says within these pages include "the most expensive pee I've ever taken," "which infection do you want?" and "my green-smoothie self." I highly recommend you read what that's all about and don't miss the chapter on hamsters. Yes, hamsters. As random as that sounds, it's part of the charm Elizabeth brings to *Percolate* by sharing her own experiences and challenges in life so that you can benefit from them. She believes that when you push fear aside, you'll find that you can "train your brain to think positively" and start to "design the life you choose." Her words, not mine.

If you think you have something to learn, keep reading. If you're at a point where you think you've got it all figured out, then that might just be when you need Elizabeth's wit and wisdom the most. And of all the books, in all the stores . . . you'll be glad you read this one.

— **Randi Siegel,**
producer, consultant, writer, and talent manager

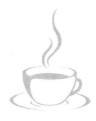

PREFACE:
LIFE IS SHORT;
LEAVE FOOTPRINTS

Did you know that almost dying leaves footprints? It does—it leaves ones the size of Big Foot's on steroids. Due to life-threatening allergic reactions, I came very close to leaving my footprints in emergency rooms during both 1998 and 1999. These experiences made me question the type of footprints I could have left behind.

Developing allergies as an adult changed my life in numerous ways . . . and nearly ended it on many occasions. After pregnancy, I developed anaphylaxis, a life-threatening reaction to food allergies. If I eat any nuts, peanuts, fish, or shellfish, I become extremely dizzy within minutes, followed by a dangerous drop in blood pressure, as well as complete digestive failure. The process of discovering which foods I was newly allergic to threatened my life on a number of occasions.

On April 10, 1998, I had my first allergic reaction while inside a coffee shop in Burnsville, Minnesota. I went there to meet my first husband, Mike, for coffee. I ate a small bag of almonds while waiting for him to arrive; and within a few minutes, I became dizzy, had severe stomach cramps, and noticed that voices started to fade as my world grew very blurry. Thinking I needed some fresh air, I stood up and made it outside to the sidewalk, but then fell to the ground and began vomiting. Thankfully, Mike arrived just in time to rush me to the hospital.

I could hardly move, so Mike had to carry me to the car. Neither of us had a clue what was happening to me. All I knew was that something was terribly wrong as I felt my energy and life rapidly fading away. I told Mike that I thought I was going to die.

Upon arrival at the ER, I was still too weak to move. The ER staff lifted me out of the car and brought me into the hospital. My blood pressure had dropped to 65/38 and was steadily decreasing. I was put on a resuscitation cart. I could hear doctors ask my husband if I had overdosed on drugs or if he knew what was wrong. He assured them that I hadn't overdosed on drugs, and that no, he hadn't a clue what had happened. While the doctors were trying to determine the reason for my rapid decline, I was unable to speak or move, and everything had become even hazier. Voices were blurred and cloudy, as forms rushed about me while numerous doctors and nurses tried desperately to save my life. My digestive system was in complete failure mode, and I had difficulty breathing. My energy was gone; everything around me faded away.

When I eventually woke up, I was hooked up to a variety of machines and drips. I felt completely overfilled with fluids the doctors had pumped into me in an attempt to save my life. Closely monitored, I spent several days on a machine that was designed to get my kidneys functioning again.

After I stabilized, the doctors and nurses informed me that it appeared I had experienced a full-blown anaphylactic reaction to some kind of food. They asked what I had eaten before the reaction, and I told them about the almonds. They warned me that if I ate almonds again, I probably wouldn't be as lucky as I was this time because allergic reactions tend to worsen after the initial exposure. The word *lucky* has stuck with me over the years. However, I spent most of the first few years following this incident feeling really angry about developing food allergies. At the time, luck never crossed my mind; I was mostly flat-out mad that I couldn't eat without fear of death.

Living with food allergies can be a challenge. I have to be extremely careful in my daily life when eating food to avoid allergens. One part of having peanut and nut allergies that is the most challenging is traveling by plane. Flying is essentially miserable and dangerous for anyone with nut allergies. Often, only peanuts are restricted on flights; however, this ban should include *all* nuts. There is nothing scarier than boarding a plane and sitting next to a person who has a bag of mixed nuts. I feel like I have a 50/50 chance of arriving at my destination versus forcing the plane into an emergency landing. I've spent years asking airlines to stop serving nuts on flights, but my pleas have mostly fallen on deaf ears. Food allergies can cause a feeling of social isolation and create anxiety around flying, going to someone's house for dinner, dining out, going to school and work, and more.

While I've had bouts of luck come into play while learning to deal with food allergies, one thing that wasn't so lucky was my first marriage. Prior to discovering my condition, my relationship with Mike was already stressed. My struggles with coming to terms with my health dealt the final blow as my marriage rapidly dissolved.

The sequence of events I'm describing is going to seem like a flurry, but out of darkness can come incredible light. As luck would have it, I met an amazing man named Peter on November 7, 1998, in New York City; and we moved to California and got married in May 1999. It was hard for my family and first husband to really understand and accept me at the time, but they largely supported my decision. They knew I needed to make a dramatic change of course, plus I had met my soul mate. In June 1999, I was visiting family in Minnesota to complete our move. I was pregnant with my third child who was due in November.

We arrived at my parents' house for a visit. Shortly after arriving, my mom offered us homemade chocolate-chip cookies. I'd eaten these delicious treats my whole life, so without much thought, I took one. After the first bite, my body immediately began to react; the cookie contained walnuts. Within minutes, I was fighting for not only my life, but also for that of our unborn son's. Instantly, my husband called 911. Due to my being pregnant, we didn't administer epinephrine. I experienced violent intestinal distress while my blood pressure dropped once again. The emergency responders worked quickly to save my life during the ambulance ride to the hospital.

Instead of me visiting my parents, they got to visit me in the hospital with our unborn son for over a week. Many tests were done to ensure that both baby Cameron and I were going to survive. We returned to our new home in Walnut Creek, California, but from that point forward, the pregnancy was difficult. I was put on anti-contraction medication and bed rest for many months. With a test to ensure Cameron's lungs were developed, labor was induced, and our baby boy was born one month early on October 29, 1999, weighing nearly seven pounds. We are both quite lucky to be here. I like to think of it as more along the lines of blessed, but I always go back to that first ER doctor telling me I was *lucky* to be alive.

> *Be grateful and reflect on the moments*
> *in life. Moments matter.*

That was 1998 and 1999, and . . . well . . . *Percolate* isn't about food allergies. Funny thing is that despite the title, this book isn't about coffee either. Actually, this is really about having courage, pushing fear aside, and making changes. It's about working with your pain, rather than resisting it. And it's about discovering how you can make the world a better place by believing in yourself and dealing with challenges by working with what you have and never giving up.

Today, I'm a mother of four boys, and no, they don't have food allergies. At the time of writing this book, our boys are 12, 14, 16, and 18, so my days are relatively free now to work and write. I didn't work very much out of the house until our youngest started school. For the most part, while home with the boys, I turned hobbies into some form of income-generating endeavor or have given back to the community. I've made more than 20,000 nut-free chocolate-chip cookies and donated them to adults and kids. Plus, I've dedicated much of my time to children's literacy.

In 2006, I became a food-allergy spokesperson for the MedicAlert Foundation and appeared on the cover of their magazine, which was mailed to over a million members. I also helped by providing them feedback on some new bracelets for children. I was featured in *One of the Gang: Nurturing the Souls of Children with Food Allergies* by Gina Clowes. These were the first instances I began to let anyone outside of my family know I had food allergies and had nearly died from them on multiple occasions. I realized that talking about my allergies could save lives and help others.

Eventually, I made the decision to reenter the world of cubicles and watercoolers. This experience changed my life. My new job was, well, unsatisfying. I say that in the nicest way possible, but it's difficult to sugarcoat the truth. The office was pretty much a workplace war zone with people constantly bickering and complaining, and it had an overall feeling of discontent. I could tell immediately that this wasn't the place for me and just knew there had to be something else I could do. I mean, here I was—a 38-year-old mother of four— longing to earn a decent income while working at home doing something where I could truly help others. Was that too much to ask? I almost began to believe it was until one day while I sat in my office contemplating my options, I finally realized what I needed to do. And thus, my company, The Best Ever You Network, was born and I resigned from my office job. Launching Best Ever You helped me start living again in the way I wanted—with even more purpose.

Fast-forward to today, and The Best Ever You Network—a community that provides unique content, creative insight, and tools through firsthand experience from a collection of diverse experts and celebrities—is a rapidly growing, leading multimedia company. We offer members the *Best Ever You* magazine and free access to Create Your Best Life, an exclusive tool designed to help people learn how to make the best choices in order to attain the *best ever* life. I always joke that I might be drinking a green smoothie for breakfast, just sitting in the kitchen in my flannel jammies, and the next moment, I'm on the phone with who knows who arranging some magazine cover or radio show. When I started this company, I had no idea that one day *The Best Ever You Show* on BlogTalkRadio would have over a million downloads. I had no idea I'd be speaking with athlete, life coach, and the ever-inspirational Gary Kobat or have the opportunity to interview Agape International founder and spiritual leader Dr. Michael Bernard Beckwith. And I certainly had no idea I'd be writing this book. There are so many "I had no idea this awesome thing would happen to me" moments as a result of making a change.

Life opens up when you shift your energy into the passions and talents that tap into your soul.

My intent in writing this book and creating The Best Ever You Network is clear: I hope to help as many people as possible live their best and most positive, peaceful lives. This book is about living with purpose and awareness to the best of your ability, and in doing so, to find community and peace within. I encourage you to value even moments of uncertainty and to leap with blind faith as you dive into your dreams. I use the word *percolate* to teach you how to filter positive changes into your life gradually and learn the importance—and benefits—of spreading this powerful way of being to others. To me, *percolating* is about working through the fear of the unknown and having the courage to savor the moments that today brings.

While reading this book (and long after you've finished it), you can turn to The Best Ever You Network (www.BestEverYou.com) daily and feel boundless energy, listen to inspiring stories from men and women from all walks of life, and find a never-ending supply of love. E-mail anyone in the community and feel the loving support, share a smile, or just know that there is always a group of friends waiting to listen to your ideas.

The Best Ever You Network is everything you need and will help you percolate happiness and success. In fact, recently I was on the phone with my mom, who said, "That company of yours has everything but the kitchen sink." My response was: "That's it! My logo is missing the kitchen sink!" We laughed. But as always, my mom was right: The Best Ever You Network does indeed have almost everything you need—well, except the kitchen sink. Who knows . . . maybe someone will send us a sink. After all, anything is possible.

Percolate and The Best Ever You Network are just what you need to become motivated to face your fears, let go of limited beliefs and thinking, and make difficult decisions to improve your life. The nine Percolate Points, which I will introduce to you shortly, will help guide you as you work your way toward becoming the person you know you can be.

Are you ready to profoundly shift your life—and have fun while doing so? Then let's start percolating!

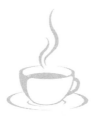

INTRODUCTION: THE PERCOLATE PROCESS

The Percolate Process™ comprises nine points that evolved from my philosophy of life, which are also grounded in my dear friend and colleague Dr. Katie Eastman's expertise in psychology and social work. With over 25 years of mental-health counseling experience, Dr. Katie is highly skilled at empowering her clients and offering them guidance through major life transitions. I'm delighted that she joins me during the "Coffee Breaks," which appear at the end of each section to help you relax, reflect, and implement what you're learning on our journey together.

◎ ◦ ◎ ◦ ◎ ◦ ◎ ◦ ◎ ◦ ◎ ◦ ◎ ◦ ◎ ◦ ◎ ◦ ◎ ◦ ◎ ◦ ◎ ◦ ◎ ◦ ◎ ◦ ◎ ◦ ◎ ◦ ◎

We developed the Percolate Points into a power-ful process to help you make meaningful, positive life changes. The catalyst of this, of course, was when I chose an "I will survive and thrive" attitude after nearly losing my life in 1998 to an allergic reaction. Motivat-ed by my two small children, I realized that moving forward required three steps: accepting this new me, being bold enough to allow my confidence to surface, and constantly reminding myself that *I am enough.*

Once I made the choice to move forward, with my best attitude and embracing my space, my thinking began to focus on how I could create my best self, and I did so by making many lifestyle changes over a period of time. I soon noticed that my own dramatic changes inspired others, and I started searching for those who were like me. Community became very important to me, and it's the reason why Best Ever You is so near and dear to my heart.

I learned firsthand that it's hard to set out to change any aspect of your lifestyle. I was even bul-lied, and encountered some very "bad brews" along the way. Undeterred, I knew that there were people with similar blends to mine, and I was determined to find them. I continued to build a community of like-minded souls. I was knocked down again with a se-rious "mocha moment"—yet another life-threatening allergic reaction that left me feeling discouraged and momentarily hopeless. However, this suddenly inspired me to brew even greater strength.

I found humor and light, and I developed incredible "self-esteam" and happiness through listening, pausing, and changing the ways in which I viewed each event that unfolded in my life. Then, I did what naturally follows in this process: I decided to use my experiences to help others. That's when I founded The Best Ever You Network to show people how to create their best brews and allow their authentic selves to filter through.

This book is about how my life experiences percolated within me and brought peace to my soul. Now, they'll hopefully inspire you to do the same. If we all percolated, then we would eventually reveal our highest purpose to help others and generate peace. Peace begins within all of us.

I'm here to help you start *percolating*. This is the process of waking up to the fact that you can make choices in every moment to make each day the best it can be. Just like brewing the perfect cup of java, there are steps that must be followed in order to achieve the life you desire. Before we embark on the journey, ask yourself the following questions:

- Is there a voice inside you saying that you want something different in life?

- Do you feel like you've been searching for something better, even if you don't know exactly what it is?

- When you hear words like *consciousness, purpose, light,* and *awaken,* do you wonder what they mean and how they apply to your life?

If you answered *yes* to any of these questions, have no fear—this book is here to provide practical and simple strategies for you to uncover your authentic self and achieve your goals! You'll become part of a growing movement to increasing compassion and transforming the world by following and adapting these nine Percolate Points into your life:

1. Allow for change to brew.

2. Choose a bolder brew.

3. Create your own best blend.

4. Grow from bean to brew.

5. Brew strength.

6. Expresso yourself.

7. Chillax and have an iced coffee.

8. Buy the next round.

9. Percolate peace.

In this fast-paced world, *Percolate* is a metaphor for how you can move forward with growing awareness, live in the present moment, and experience greater joy and peace. It's a way to get you to:

- Wake up to what is possible without losing sight of the simple and practical things that already exist.

- Let your heart and mind brew powerful ideas so that your spirit floats to the top like the foam on your latte.

- Live your best life and thrive.

Most important, *Percolate* helps you to never give up on living your best life every day. So, grab a cup of your favorite joe, put your feet up, and let your heart's desire surface. Ah, can you taste the magic as you bring the authentic, best you to the world?

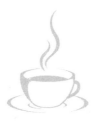

LET'S STIR THINGS UP

I hope you're sitting down on your comfy couch or in your favorite spot in your coffee shop and are excited to start percolating with me. Whether you're in your jammies or a suit, let's have a chat about the Percolate Process. The goal is to wake you up and stir your thoughts.

In order to help you make real improvements in your life, I want your Percolate experience to be empowering. In other words, we're practicing meaningful, positive change. There are certain things in life that are consistent and reliable; however, Mother Nature is always reminding us that nothing stays the same. The challenge rests with how we manage change and when we should begin the change process.

The following are some simple questions and principles to consider as you follow the Percolate Process. Just keep these in mind as you percolate. Dr. Katie and I will be checking in with you through the Coffee Breaks between the Percolate Points to help keep you on track and make this as easy and fun as possible.

Are you ready? Let's get started!

How do you make meaningful, positive changes? How many times have you decided that you wanted to improve some aspect of your life but then gave up within a few days of starting to do so? Why do most of us do this, and how can we avoid the stumbling blocks that prevent us from maintaining whatever changes we make? The Percolate Process is focused on small, incremental changes over time. I want you to relax into this experience and consider a new aspect of your vision for your best life every time you pick up a cup of joe.

How do you implement the changes you desire despite challenges? In spite of your greatest intentions, daily life brings the unpredictable, and obstacles beyond your control can sabotage your best efforts. Sometimes the coffee just tastes bad, or, even worse, the coffeepot breaks! What should you do during those times? Pause, think creatively, and consider what can be done to maintain what is most important while asking yourself what you might need to let go. Throughout this process, you must ask yourself what *can* you do rather than what *can't* you do.

What are your values? Every day you make decisions—lots of them! You're constantly having to decide what you're going to eat, what you say to others, how you behave, how you spend your time, and so on. These choices are all based on what's important to you. Therefore, when making these decisions, it's necessary to ask yourself, *What do I really care about, and what do I value the most?* As you reflect and percolate, you may realize that you discover new values. Embrace them! This is all part of the Percolate Process.

What are your beliefs? What we believe is what we think about all day, every day. When you change your thoughts, you change your behavior. Be clear about what you believe to be true, and challenge those beliefs as you go through this process. Change is not just about behavior; it's also about the thoughts that direct the behavior.

What areas of your life do you want to make changes in? This may change every day, several times a day. Keep a Percolate journal, be flexible, try new things, be open to new ideas, and most of all . . . *percolate!*

Can you give yourself the time to make genuine changes? Pause as you engage the Percolate Process, and allow changes to happen slowly. There's a reason why I wrote a whole book on this process! It takes time, it takes reflection, and it takes a whole lot of daily coffee brewing to live your best life each day. The Percolate Process is a lifestyle, not a quick fix. If you really like a latte, then wait for it. Don't settle for instant decaf.

As we begin percolating together, I encourage you to do a self-inventory and take a close look at your life. Ask yourself the following questions:

- *What footprints am I leaving?*

- *Am I making the world a better place? In what ways? If not, what's holding me back?*

- *How am I living my day-to-day life? How do I feel most days?*

- *Are there people in my life who have my back, and vice versa?*

It may take you 5 minutes, 30 days, 3 years, or 99 steps in whatever direction to get you to your goals. Remember that how long or how many steps you have to take doesn't matter—the most important thing is *getting* there . . . and you will if you focus and percolate with me. And when you do so, you'll even enhance and inspire the lives of those around you. Search with me for something better, even if you don't know exactly what that is. When our lives touch, our goal is that we all become our best, authentic selves as a result.

Percolate Point #1

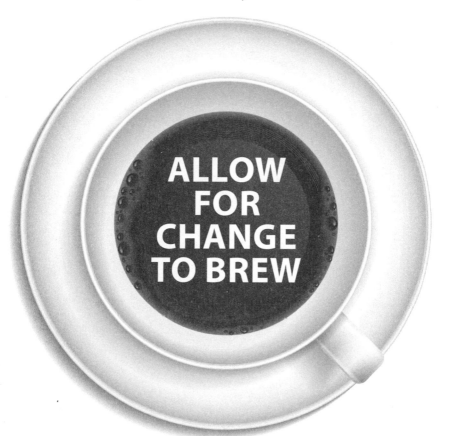

ALLOW
FOR
CHANGE
TO BREW

Discovering Your Inner Aardvark and Platypus

Life is full of choices about how to live and, for some, it includes choosing life itself. In August 2004, my kids, husband, and I moved across the country to Portland, Maine. Prior to the move, we'd spent months trying to decide whether we should move to Maine or Minnesota. Although my parents were living in Minnesota, and it would've been nice to be close to them, we opted for Maine because my husband's job offer there was a bit better. Besides, we figured my parents would love to visit, eat lobster, and take in the gorgeous scenery.

Sounds like a great plan, right? Unfortunately, however, life had something else in mind. . . .

On December 18, 2004, with my home still un-packed and boxes everywhere, I found myself boarding a plane from Maine to Minnesota, as my 60-year-old dad had suffered a stroke. He had collapsed in the living room of my parents' house the day before. My brother Shane had, by sheer luck, just learned the symptoms of a stroke a few days earlier. He recognized the signs immediately and called an ambulance. Shortly after the stroke, my dad suffered a brain hemorrhage that was devastating and called for extreme life-saving mea-sures, including a barbiturate-induced coma.

I spent much of 2005 flying back and forth between Maine and Minnesota while my dad fought for his life. During this experience, I also discovered that I need-ed to help keep my mom healthy. She was completely devastated and stressed out, even sobbing in her sleep. I'd heard about instances of longtime married couples dying together: when one spouse becomes critically ill and dies, the other dies of a broken heart at the same time or shortly after. Having been married for over 30 years, my mother was a prime candidate for this. It felt like we would lose our mom, too, if our dad died or just from the sheer stress from watching him suffer. So my siblings and I tried to do everything in our power to prevent that from happening.

This was an intense period of ups and downs and near-death moments. During this time, my family members and I bonded with the doctors and nurses on staff. My dad's room was plastered with photographs of his children and grandchildren—the positive energy was abundant. It was clear that my dad loved movies, basketball, and other sports, too, as that energy was present in the room. We worked hard to keep my dad's morale up by reminding him of all the things he had left to do in the world: attending weddings, meeting future grandchildren, and so on.

However, at one point, the cardiologist gathered the entire family around. This seasoned professional cried as he informed us that he had done everything in his power to save my dad's life, but he feared the outlook was grim. Everyone in the room could tell he felt intense responsibility for keeping our dad alive, but it seemed so very hopeless. Despite his prediction, we found ourselves offering him hugs during this sad moment. In the midst of this most difficult conversation, the doctor mentioned that he would love to play basketball with Dad and all of us because we just seemed like such a cool, loving family. We cried. We prayed. We stayed positive and never gave up.

I flew back and forth for most of the year. On one occasion with my dad still in a coma, when things seemed completely desperate, while getting ready to return to Minnesota, I found myself alternating between crying and sobbing as I packed black funeral clothes in my suitcase. Then on that miraculous day in the middle of 2005, the phone rang. The call was completely out of the blue.

"Hello," the extremely weak, barely recognizable, and faint voice said, "It's me, Dad. I love you."

Caught completely off guard, with the coat of a black suit in hand, it took me a second to grasp what I'd just heard. *It was my dad's voice.* I couldn't believe it—my dad was speaking to me! My mom then took the phone because Dad was speaking to me while on a ventilator, a feat that is nearly impossible to do. When he woke from the coma, he'd requested to make a phone call to me. Just typing this makes me feel the warmth and abundance of gratitude.

My dad was alive—and, better yet, he not only came out of the coma, but for some miraculous reason that none of us really completely understands, my dad also had most of his faculties in order. His memory was perfect, and he could move. His speech was faded and weak, but it was clear to us all he would survive.

I packed brighter clothes and immediately flew back to Minnesota. Even today, it is quite difficult to remove that image of my dad when he was so ill from my mind. Many of us kids had nightmares and illnesses of our own that year because of the stress.

One thing I learned from my parents during this experience is the incredible strength they both showed. During this ICU stay, my dad was on a ventilator and for the most part unable to speak. We all discovered that years ago, our mom and dad had worked out a code to use in case of a situation such as this. If either of them became unable to speak, they promised to blink twice if the sick person could hear and squeeze a hand if they felt extreme pain. Throughout Dad's critical care stay in the hospital, he and my mom used this code much too often for the amount of tears I could cry. It's certainly a code of strength I'll never forget.

Months passed while Dad received treatment at the rehab center. We didn't know whether he would ever fully recover the use of his eyesight, speech, or hearing. There were some extremely dicey moments with fevers, involuntary hiccups, and just overall extreme weakness. These were things that set back the progress one hopes to make in a rehab center. Thankfully, as he began to recover, Dad gradually regained his strength and voice. There were no major issues to the extent of needing to go back to the ICU or hospital, but plenty of close calls and trying moments where continued will to survive was needed.

One day, rather unexpectedly, a gray-haired, spunky older nurse came into his room and told my dad that it was time to get him ready to go to speech therapy. My dad is about 6'4", well over 280 pounds, and at the time, he was in pretty rough shape. I know the last thing on his mind was speech therapy, but as many of us know, cooperation is important while in the hospital. It took several people what seemed like forever to properly maneuver him and his many cords and bottles in order to transfer him from his hospital bed into a wheelchair. He was already exhausted from that process, and despite his lack of energy and enthusiasm, my dad went along for the ride.

Now, my dad is a very smart man. Little did we know, but he was going to teach us a *new* code. The nurse who wheeled Dad down to his speech pathologist spoke to him in a gentle, baby-talk voice. She asked my dad to say the first word that came to mind when she said a letter of the alphabet. Naturally, she started with *A*. I suppose the nurse expected Dad to say *at* or *and,* words typical from a patient who had suffered such a severe stroke.

Dad looked over at us, rolled his eyes, and said, "Aardvark." My translation of Dad's code: "Do you think I am so debilitated that I've lost my mind, too?"

Dad, draped in fashionable hospital garb, exhausted, barely fitting in the wheelchair, and having now been in the hospital for months, was about to recite the preschool alphabet for all of us in a new way.

The next letter was *B*.

"Benevolence," he whispered. Mom and I giggled. Then came *C*.

"Courage."

And *D*.

"Definitely determination," he said, smiling.

I'm fairly certain my dad's word selection for the letter *F* was, well, not appropriate for this book. We blamed that response on the drugs. For *M*, Dad chose "movies," and from out of nowhere came "platypus" for the letter *P*. The therapy continued through to the letter *Z*.

Although the nurse was astounded by my dad's vocabulary choices, Mom and I weren't surprised at all. My dad's mantra has always been *I can and I will*. Listening to him utter these words brought hope, courage, and laughter. Despite the trauma of a stroke and four brain surgeries, Dad maintained his wit and humor; it was his way of telling us he was going to be okay.

Thinking about the words *I can't* help me realize that our life experiences teach us what we are capable of achieving. It's easy to lose track of our successes when life becomes overwhelming. Eventually, we start to feel like we can't do something we love, or it's too late to be that writer we've always wanted to be, or that famous painter, or the adventurer longing to visit the rain forests of Costa Rica. We get stuck in the words *I can't* and give up on these dreams.

This is where percolating comes in and perhaps my favorite word will soon become yours, too.

When someone tells me they *can't* do something, I immediately think about my dad's experiences at the rehab center. I long to take the *can't-sayer* on a field trip to this inspiring institute just to show what can be done when you change *can't* to *can*. We spent months in this amazing facility, wondering if my dad would ever speak, walk, or see again. My mom and I would go on hospital walks during those bleak and desperate moments. While we wandered the mazes of halls, we'd gaze upon and admire the artwork displayed on the walls. Not until we closely examined the art did we realize who the artists were—blind people painting from memory, children whose limbs were deformed due to the effects of thalidomide, paralyzed patients painting with their mouth, feet, or even eyelashes. These incredible creations inspired us. They weren't just your average works of art—no, these images on the walls were miracles made from determination and the unwillingness to say *I can't*.

You can. Whenever my mom or I experience a challenging moment in our lives, we talk a lot about what we witnessed at the rehab center. My mom recently called to tell me that one of her friends asked her to speak at her funeral when she dies. I thought that was a strange request because the friend seemed young—just my mom's age. Mom reminded me that many people her age start thinking about their death, especially when they begin to have more serious health problems. Her friend had just been diagnosed with diabetes.

Rather than agree to the request, Mom surprised her friend by suggesting some dietary and exercise changes to help manage her illness and prolong her life. Despite this newfound knowledge, my mom's friend struggled with the diet changes and felt quite sad and hopeless.

I see this as an opportunity for her friend to awaken, to feel love and compassion for herself, and to begin to make changes. The pain and sadness provide an opportunity, and maybe even a chance, to become a medical wake-up call. Mom offered to help her friend adhere to the new diet and exercise regime, and she ended their conversation by assuring her that there would be plenty of time to discuss her funeral plans.

In contrast, my mom has another friend who is 83 years old. My mom's friend is so excited about her daughter's second wedding that she keeps sending my mom pictures on her cell phone of the new dresses that she is considering wearing to the special occasion, as well as jewelry and shoe choices. In fact, her friend has gone on a diet in preparation for her daughter's big day. Now, *that's* living. After telling me about her two friends, Mom said, "You can spend all of your time dying, or you can live. It's your choice." I don't know about you, but I choose to *live*.

Let's face it: For the most part, life isn't predictable. I know—that just seems so unfair, but since we have no way of knowing when or where we will draw our last breath, it's important to begin embracing life *now*. If you're reading this, *smile*. You can even giggle or laugh. After all, you're *alive*. Some mornings, it might not be that easy to just roll out of bed full of gratitude, plant those feet on the floor, and feel tremendous love for the day ahead. I get it; I'm usually fumbling around for my glasses that have fallen on the floor or socks that I've kicked off in the middle of the night, but if you think about the alternative, it makes the task a whole lot easier. You might have to learn how to do it, but it's an important lesson to master.

Here's an idea: Try spending some time reviewing your day and giving thanks for all the great moments—and yes, even for the not-so-great ones. Do this each night before you fall asleep, and ask yourself the following:

- Are you able to maintain a positive sense of yourself?

- Are you still positive to those around you under these wearisome circumstances?

How do you give thanks for a difficult moment? Perhaps it makes you appreciate the good ones all the more. This practice becomes especially important when life gets tough and throws you a curve, twist, or fireball.

Despite any challenge, with thought and reflection, you *can* focus on the positive and not drown in a pool of negativity, stress, or anxiety.

Percolate.
Be determined.

Bold Beginnings

The alphabet is one of the first things we learn in life and one of the first ways we express ourselves as children. From ABC songs to Dr. Seuss books, there are all sorts of games we played as kids to learn our letters.

If you have children, think of the time invested in teaching them to write, memorize, recite, and learn the alphabet. It's the foundation of our language, so much so that when I say the letter *A*, most people would respond with the word *apple* and not *aardvark*. Well, my dad inspired me to play a new alphabet game. Let's say that the first word that comes to mind for the letter *A* isn't apple. What if it's *attitude?* Would it be as catchy?

Could your brain reeducate itself to think of *attitude* as the most dominant *A* word? What if we taught our kids this type of vocabulary from the start? What if we used those precious hours of early learning and taught life lessons using the alphabet?

The first step is to realize that the ABCs of life begin with positive thinking. You can retrain your brain to think positively; it's as important as learning the alphabet. Consider the words you use daily or even moment to moment, and think about what you say around others. Before you do this though, it's important to stop believing that everyone else has it better than you. You know it when you think it—it's someone who has a cleaner car, more cash in the bank, a bigger shoe collection, a higher-paying job, a book deal, a better body, or whatever you might perceive is true of someone else's life. You think that everyone around the world has a perfect life . . . except you! There are days when you might catch yourself glancing at the marks on your kitchen walls thinking the house across the street is perfectly unscathed.

But whose reality are you really seeing? Upon closer inspection, you'll likely discover that nobody has the perfect life, and for the cleanest, best waxed car that ever existed, there is most likely a crumb or two somewhere inside. Therefore, it's important to focus on yourself and *only* yourself with respect to your life and to *only* evaluate how you are doing in it. I keep the word *perfect* out of the vocabulary at Best Ever You. After all, it says Best Ever You, not Perfect Ever You.

So let's start creating our own Alphabet of Life. Are you brewing a pot of sad, depressing, or angry words; or are you brewing a colorful, positive, energy-rich vocabulary? The words you say to yourself affect how you feel and how you behave. Just as the alphabet is the foundation of our language, how we express ourselves begins with our thoughts.

Throughout the Percolate Process, I'll be asking you to reflect and interact with me as you *percolate,* and now is the perfect time to encourage you to begin keeping a Percolate journal. Let's make your personal Alphabet of Life the first entry in your journal. I'll start by sharing my own alphabet. The following is a list of words I use daily. They're part of my Alphabet of Life because they bring a smile to my face during trying times, inspire me to be my best self, and give me strength.

Elizabeth's Alphabet of Life

A	Acceptance	Awaken	Advocate	Altruism	Aardvark
B	Best	Believe	Benevolence	Be	Beauty
C	Courage	Compassion	Change	Choices	Consistency
D	Do	Decisive	Dream	Dare	Determination
E	Educate	Elegance	Excellence	Enjoy	Empower
F	Faith	Footprints	Fortitude	Funny	Fairy Godmother
G	Grace	Giving	Goodness	Gratitude	Gentle
H	Health	Hamster	Heart	Humor	Happyometer
I	Intuition	Introspection	Integrity	Inspire	Imagine
J	Joy	Joyology	Jog	Joke	Journey
K	Keys	Knowing	Kindness	Kindle	Knowledge
L	Love	Laugh	Learn	Live	Listen
M	Motivate	Mission	Mentor	Music	Map
N	No!	Noble	Notable	Necessary	Natural
O	Open-minded	Opportunities	Ouch!	Open	Obligations
P	Percolate	Platypus	Purpose	Passion	Peace
Q	Quiet	Quest	Question	Quirky	Queue
R	Relax	Read	Remember	Reexamine	Recharge
S	Smile	Serious	Success	Stop	Silence
T	Tolerant	Teach	Test	Try	Tact
U	Unburden	Unlearn	Unbridle	Upfront	Understanding

V	Vision	Value	Vacation	Vibration	Versatile
W	Wisdom	Weight	Wellness	Wonder	Wit
X	Xenia	Xenolith	Xanadu	eXciting	Xxoo
Y	Yes!	You	Youth	Yield	Yearn
Z	Ziggle	Zaggle	Zip	Zeal	Zest

Are you ready? It's your turn now! Reach for your Percolate journal, and write down words that give you courage, make you laugh, and motivate you to move forward in life. Start creating your own Alphabet of Life.

Percolate.
Be positive.

Time for a New Flavor

What's next after you explore your language and your life? Countless self-help books tell you to just accept yourself, boost your self-esteem, and on and on . . . yet negative chatter continues to plague most people. Although this book isn't a magic pill, I hope that the reflections in the previous chapters help you recognize your strengths and discover areas for improvement. I also hope you're starting to feel motivated and inspired to make changes. I won't sugarcoat it—the path of self-improvement can be challenging.

Do you tend to whine, gripe, or complain? Or maybe you're a self-loving, self-appreciating, and accepting soul. No one prances around in Happy Land

24/7, but you can learn to move more easily toward happiness and find it in the strangest places—just as my family did in that rehab center in Minnesota.

Let's begin with the whines, gripes, and complaints. You know the most common ones: "I'm fat!" or "I never have enough money!" Perhaps 99.9 percent of us live with these words on the tips of our tongues. After having four children, I can safely say that I was never one of those gals who put on her skinny jeans a few weeks after giving birth. Years of up-and-down weight gain and having a baby every other year for eight years does a number on the body. I used to step on the scale and cry. Oh, the rivers I've cried! So I made an executive decision nearly two years ago to hide my scale. This was the first time in my life when I didn't weigh myself nearly every day—and sometimes twice a day. Keep in mind that I wasn't really doing much fitness- or food-wise either in order to get the numbers down. I was simply stepping on the scale, feeling sorry for myself, and wishing to be thin.

The result of hiding the scale was amazing. I replaced my daily internal chatter that chided me for my weight with a daily reminder of how happy I was with myself. Am I any heavier now than I was before I hid the scale? No. Once I relaxed about my weight, I became both happier and thinner. *Did I mention thinner?*

I recently lovingly reclaimed my scale. Personally, I'd like to invent a new scale exclusively for women. This special scale will have buttons on the side to press: "Lie to Me" lists your weight as ten pounds less, and "Happy Holidays" lists your weight as ten pounds heavier but sings holiday songs in the background and gently reminds you to take it easy on the cookies. While there could be many other buttons, I'd add the "Keep up the Great Work!" setting. This one weighs you as two to three pounds lighter—like most of us used to set our scales anyway—and then it reminds you to keep up the great eating and fitness habits.

However, today, instead of weighing myself with disgust when my pants are snug, I focus on the positive feelings I have of being healthy again—both mentally and physically. I now realize that I am here, I am valuable, and my life is meaningful and cherished regardless of what the scale says back to me. I've learned to make small, positive changes in other areas that bother me, and as a result, I feel relief as that internal chatter disappears.

Try to put this into practice by saying the following affirmations to yourself daily:

I accept myself. I love myself. I accept those around me. I am compassionate.

I accept my faults, flaws, and mistakes.
I am worth it.
I appreciate my life.
I advocate for my beliefs, my rights, and myself.
I lovingly take care of myself.

Feel free to add your own affirmations, and jot them down in your journal.

Accepting What You Can't Change

It's also important to accept that there are just some things you can't change. There are poems, stories, and songs written about acceptance. No matter how hard you wish, try, or hope to wake up one day and have whatever it is magically resolved or removed from your life, sometimes it just won't happen and you need to accept it.

You may not know this, but the AARP starts sending out information when you turn 50 years old. You can react by either burning the welcome packet or by taking advantage of the many discounts the organization offers. With age comes wisdom and rewards for the wisdom. It truly is a gift if you choose to view it that way. The AARP magazine has been arriving at our house for my husband, and I can tell you that it completely freaked me out when it first showed up in our mailbox. It was like we'd been officially declared old. Then the blessing appeared when we discovered the joys of age . . . hotel discounts!

However, some things just are what they are and will be what they will be. You can't change your age. You can't change your height. You can't change your DNA—well, maybe with a good scientist or toxic cloud, but you can't change what something truly is. You can lie and fake it, but you can't change it.

I know this woman who, at around age 55, went for a major facelift to remove ten years from her appearance. Her heart was still 55 years old, her feet were still 55 years old, her hands were still 55 years old, and her bones were still 55 years old—she was still 55 years old. I refer to a set of her photos from this time as the Botox pictures because her eyes are so wide open and she has the strangest facial expressions. The surgery didn't really remove years. Instead, it taught this woman a valuable lesson: that beauty and self-esteem come from inside. She discovered that she was already beautiful because she was such a wonderful person. She is now closer to 70 years old and couldn't care less how many wrinkles she has. Her family cherishes each and every one.

You make a choice how you view what you can't change. You can whine for a minute, choose to accept what you can't change, and then remind yourself that there's a different opportunity available. Aging is one of those things you can't change. What you can change, however, is how you think about aging.

Sometimes a health crisis or accident causes us to have a permanent change. I think of my friend Sarah Bazey from Minneapolis, Minnesota. Sarah is a Harvard Business School graduate and the owner and president of Simplex Construction Supplies, Inc. In 1994, she chartered a helicopter to survey a concrete paving project for which her company supplied construction materials. Sadly, the flight ended in a horrific crash. Sarah suffered third-degree burns over 40 percent of her body when the helicopter exploded. She went on to endure 15 surgeries, 18 months of therapy, and countless medical procedures. Today, she proudly serves as vice president of the National Board of Trustees for the Phoenix Society for Burn Survivors, a national nonprofit organization dedicated to empowering burn victims through support programs, education, and advocacy.

I came across Sarah and her story one day while reading about the various contestants from the Mrs. International website. For the past several years, I have interviewed a contestant from this pageant because of the cause-based focus of the competition, meaning that the ladies involved have to have a social platform of discussion during their year. On that particular day, I saw a contestant with the most beautiful emerald eyes. There was a look of determination in her that was different from the other contestants. The woman was none other than Sarah Bazey, Mrs. Minnesota International. Upon reading her story, I asked her to be a guest on *The Best Ever You Show*. As she shared her story with our listeners, we could all tell she had been through hell and back. She had gone from being a beautiful blonde with gorgeous skin to a disfigured, somewhat unrecognizable burn survivor. It gave me chills when she described how she asked for a mirror after the accident to "see how bad it was."

Sarah said that while she was mortified by the reflection of her face, she could see her eyes, and she knew that she was going to be okay—yes, those same determined eyes that drew my attention on the website. She told us that at one point during rehab, things were so miserable that she just lost it. She had a total meltdown, but after 30 minutes of complete release, her pity party was over, and she realized that all of her energy was needed to focus on healing and moving forward. Alive and with recoverable circumstances, that is exactly what she did. It was very clear to me that she would absolutely be the next Mrs. International. I asked her to come back on the show if she won.

She kept her promise. In July 2012, Sara was crowned Mrs. International, and in September, she was once again a guest on the show. This was her message:

> As a burn survivor, it is an honor to wear the Mrs. Minnesota International crown and share my story with others who may struggle with scars or disfigurement. We can never be reminded enough about the beauty that lies within each of us. Life often has a way of challenging us when we least expect it. How we choose to respond to the challenge, what we learn from the experience, and whether or not we help others by sharing our story is up to us.[1]

Now it's your turn! Grab your Percolate journal, and write down your answers to the following:

- List five things that bother you about yourself that you can't change.

- List at least five ways that you're going to start accepting what you can't change.

Percolate.
Be accepting.

A Pocket Full
of Change

It takes courage to make changes in our lives. Our habits are familiar and have become comfortable behaviors we wake up to every day. Change takes courage because we are required to step outside the box and shake things up a bit. Some of our relationships even become like a pair of comfortable slippers that have grown worn and in need of repair. By reading this book, you've made a choice to find the nerve to create a life for yourself filled with happiness, self-love, self-worth, joy, compassion, and being your best. You've chosen what has meaning to you and what doesn't.

There are so many variables that create change in our lives—some more drastic than others. On a day-to-day basis, this change is something we can set at our own pace, but sometimes our lives change in an instant because of unforeseen events. Wonderful things can show up, such as falling in love, receiving a promotion, or winning the lottery, but there are also changes that can cause great shifts or create challenges we are required to deal with. They all create instantaneous change—ready or not.

The loss of a loved one is one of the most difficult changes to deal with. For instance, my friend Debra Oakland received a phone call one Sunday morning at 5:00 A.M. informing her that her 21-year-old son had been killed in a car accident while he was in Canada. Debra told me the following:

> I could not comprehend what my husband was saying. We were in shock, such a strange feeling . . . so foreign to us both. If I sat still, I needed to move. If I moved about, I needed to find a quiet space. We ended up attending an event we'd planned to go to that morning. We didn't know what else to do. My son was in another country, and we had to get through the day. This event was instrumental in dealing with the beginning of our grief. The subject [of the lecture] was the loss of children. It is a very

long story I will share another time, but I want you to know that this event was such an unexpected blessing in a time of great sadness.[1]

You never know who or what will show up to support you in your time of need. Debra has gone on to become a courage advocate and helps others on a daily basis. She has also written the book *Living in Courage: A Spiritual Oasis for Overcoming Life's Biggest Challenges* to share her story and help others.

Another example of the tremendous courage it takes to become an advocate in the face of an unexpected tragedy comes from the Hom family. Living with food allergies is a real challenge, one that is very near and dear to my heart. Brian and Kathy Hom lost their son due to an allergic reaction from food. Brian James Hom II, known as BJ, turned 18 on June 25, 2008, and had just graduated from high school. The family took a vacation to celebrate these two milestones and traveled to Cabo San Lucas, Mexico, in July. Brian and Kathy arrived at the hotel with BJ and his two younger brothers in the late afternoon. They were hungry, but the restaurants were closed except for the buffet. After depositing the luggage in their rooms, they all went down to eat. After dinner, the setting sun was beautiful, so they decided to take a beach walk and check out the swimming pool at the resort. While on their exploration, BJ complained to his father about a sore throat. Brian had no idea that this would be the last conversation he would ever have with his son.[2]

They walked to the gift shop to buy cough drops, and as BJ took one, he told his mom that he didn't feel well and needed to go back to the hotel room. Just before entering the elevator, BJ became extremely ill, so they sat down in the lobby while Kathy ran to the front desk for help. Unknowingly, Brian and his two younger sons had gone to the arcade. A hotel guest ran into the arcade and informed Brian that there was an emergency. They all ran to the lobby area and found BJ gasping for air. His face was pale, and his lips had turned blue. Although there was no doctor on the premises at the time, everyone tried to help because they thought the cough drop had gotten stuck in BJ's throat. When the paramedics came, they attempted resuscitation and thought BJ was going to be okay because he was finally breathing. However, a little later when the doctor arrived to check on BJ, this promising 18-year-old had died.

The family felt as if their hearts had been torn out of their chests. They were overcome with shock and grief. Unable to leave Mexico for three days added to their pain. Brian's younger son had a skin reaction on his face after BJ passed away, which prompted them to ask if there were peanuts in any of the food. The restaurant told them that the chocolate mousse dessert had traces of peanuts in it.

Enduring this type of tragedy takes tremendous courage for any family, but to then direct their grief toward helping others is almost unimaginable. This amazing family teaches us that when faced with such a tragedy, our grief, anger, frustration, or whatever feelings we have can motivate us to help others avoid a similar situation. The Hom family has taken the loss of BJ and turned it into something positive. Since BJ's death, Brian and Kathy have been raising awareness about the dangers of food allergies and educating people to protect themselves and their children. Brian is also a member of the board of directors for the Food Allergy & Anaphylaxis Connection Team (FAACT). The Homs are now food-allergy advocates, using many avenues to help save the lives of others with the hope that no one will ever suffer a loss like their family has.

These examples of amazing courage can inspire all of us to take whatever steps we need to make changes in our lives. If they can do it, so can you! Even in the face of unimaginable loss, you have to be willing to ask yourself, *How can I live my best life?* Without making this resolve, healing can't happen and life can't change. Let others' stories motivate you to make whatever changes will make your life better. You don't have to wait for tragedy to strike. Rather, remember that life is short and unpredictable; make changes now, and have the courage to be your best.

Direct your thoughts in a positive direction, and keep seeking what is meaningful to you. Make it your intention to take one action daily. Changing new habits will multiply in effects—just like collecting pennies eventually leads to saving dollars. Remember what it felt like to be a child when every penny you placed in your piggy bank filled you with the anticipation of what it could be like when your bank was completely full? Imagine you're creating your life in the same way—into a real-life piggy bank full of all the wonderful changes you wish to make. Each small change is like those pennies, and every time you take a step in a new direction, you move with courage. Take those steps; grab those imaginary pennies; and replace the old, familiar behaviors with something positive and meaningful.

Percolate.
Be courageous.

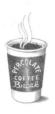

Coffee Break with Elizabeth and Dr. Katie

A Small Sip of Change

It's Elizabeth and Dr. Katie to check in on how you're doing. Are you starting to *percolate?* Have you begun thinking about making—dare we utter the word—*changes?* Most people run for cover at the mere mention of the word. Or better yet, they'll race away in search of vast quantities of chocolate. Change makes people sweat, gag, or feel a whole lot of stress and anxiety. Why? Because we get used to what is familiar. We find comfort in routine and what we can expect. Like our shabby old bathrobe with years of coffee stains that we've held on to for too long, we like what we know and fear what we don't.

If you hear yourself talking in *who, what, where, when, why,* and *will* mode, listen carefully to yourself because change might be brewing. Have you caught yourself saying any of the following?

- *What if I quit my job?*

- *What will happen if I move?*

- *Will people make fun of me?*

- *Will I be okay?*

- *When will I resolve this issue?*

- *Where will I be?*

- *Why should I do that?*

- *Who will I meet?*

- *What will happen to me when I make the change?*

- *Where, when, and how will I know if I'll be okay?*

If you've had any of those thoughts, then welcome to a big, whopping dose of *change.* Change happens all around you, all of the time. You can't control much of it, and that lack of control is what causes people to fear the unknown. Welcome ambiguity. It's fuzzy. You might not be able to see clearly, and perhaps you're afraid or angry because you can't control the situation.

When we set out to make changes in our lives, there are times when we think that we'd really like to upgrade to that bright yellow bathrobe—but, *Oh jeez, what if I get coffee stains on this new one?* So instead of trying to get used to the new, we go back to our old coffee-stained and comfortable robe. Instead of trying a green smoothie, we stick to our regular bacon-and-egg breakfast. It takes a lot of trying on the new over and over before we feel comfortable with the change. Eventually we realize that the coffee has been sitting on the burner for too long, and we finally pitch the old robe and embrace the new one.

Remember to keep in mind there are some things that can't change, and you must learn to accept them as they are. Next time you go into a coffee shop, make sure you're drinking freshly *percolated* coffee. That's what you deserve.

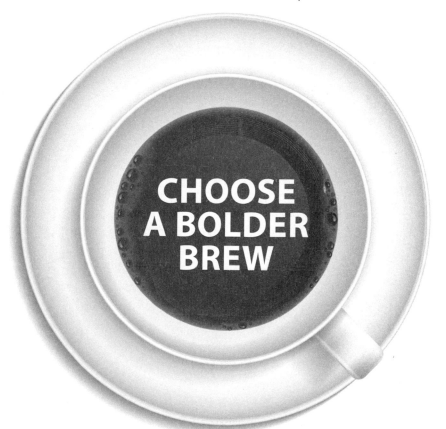

CHOOSE
A BOLDER
BREW

What Would Betty White Do?

Change can leave you feeling indecisive, scared, and even stressed. It's scary to move out of your safe *hamster zone* (we'll talk about this later) and into the unknown of doing something different. So, in comes actress Betty White. It's no secret that I'm a big fan. Betty doesn't know it, but anyone who hangs out with me is well aware that she's one of my idols. To me, Betty is fearless, funny, and real. She's a perfect example of percolating the best cup of coffee around. She inspires me with her class and humor.

In times of indecision, I often ask myself WWBWD: What Would Betty White Do? Would she choose a cup of the serious Sumatra or go for a lighter New England blend? The answer is clear and always the same: Betty would probably laugh and go light! I love and appreciate that she doesn't take herself too seriously. She exudes a level of confidence and courage that I constantly aspire to achieve. You'll often see me tweet: "In any time of indecision or confusion, ask yourself #WWBWD? 99.9 percent of the time you'll have your answer." I really do think that laughter is the best stress crusher. I strongly believe that we should just be ourselves and be hilarious doing it. By doing so, we show the world that we're confident and comfortable being who we are.

So the next time you're feeling overly stressed, see if you can find a glimmer of humor in it, and ask yourself WWBWD. I promise you that if you just stop and ask yourself this question, nine times out of ten, you'll laugh or have distracted yourself from the problem. This doesn't mean you shouldn't take what is happening seriously. It really just means to try to put things into perspective and keep the stress in check. If finding the right dress for an event puts you straight into heart-palpitation mode, for example, go pick out the craziest, ugly dress you can find at the store, try it on, and have a laugh at yourself. If you get crazed every time you try to put on false eyelashes, like I do, find a few stuck to your hair during an important event once or twice in your lifetime, and have a crazy good chuckle.

It's amazing how freeing it is to be able to laugh at yourself. No longer do you worry about what others think, but instead, you gain the self-assurance to feel that you can handle anything that comes your way. Once you achieve this feeling, you gain the ability to dream big. Remember Walt Disney's wise words: "If you can dream it, you can do it." Well, it's true— you can! In fact, to make changes and better choices in your life, dream about them first. I say dream and keep dreaming with a dash of determination, decisiveness, and sense of humor thrown in. Reach up and set the bar higher with everything you do. Commitment and consistency help dreams become reality. Stay the course and never give up. The journey getting to your dreams will be nothing like what you imagined. In fact, you'll discover that what you've dreamed actually takes on many forms along the way. However, the most important thing is to remember to stay the course, hold steady, and embrace opportunities.

Taking the First Step

Let's take that first step to achieving your goals. Remember, choose the lighter blend of life and stay true to yourself as you begin the voyage. I know you have the courage to do it, and *you* know you have it. Grab your Percolate journal and reflect on these questions:

- It's decision time: Will your goals stay a dream, or will they become a reality?

- What factors will help you decide to make a huge change?

- Will you feel better?

- What will be mended?

- What will get broken?

- What can you live with?

- What can you live without?

- Have you evaluated the pros and cons?

- Do you feel comfortable knowing what you're getting into?

There is one more level of courage, determination, and self-confidence that is necessary before taking that first step. It's a leap of faith! Having the courage to change ultimately relies on the faith you have in yourself and your ability to cope with whatever arises. There are no right or wrong answers when making the decision to change; there are no guarantees that one option will ultimately be the best. That's why a variety of choices will eventually make the process better. We create our best change.

Percolate.
Be decisive.

Taking Inventory

I will never forget the period between 2006 and 2008. I was feeling stuck in a job I strongly disliked, and although my father was continuing to make progress in his health, overall, he was still very weak. My brother Justin survived a brutal attack, and my mom was being treated at the Mayo Clinic for leukoplakia, which was probably caused by stress. And to top it all off nicely, I continued to do battle with food allergies and reactions. Challenges like a flat tire on a car or dinner burned in the oven felt like they were all that were needed to add to the stress that could create a robust blend of massive anxiety. There were nights when I had to sleep propped up after downing antacids because of the pain from heartburn.

Stress is a killer.

I felt like there had to be a way to acquire harmony and create a baseline of peacefulness to my life. And if I did that, then maybe I could focus on gratitude. Finding strength within became the key to doing this.

Instead of focusing on the problems, I brought all of my passions, talents, energy, and problem-solving skills together to create and develop The Best Ever You Network. I implemented some new beliefs and practices in my own life and took it a step further by inviting columnists to share their expert advice on health, well-being, relationships, work, success, and other topics in order to help people live their Best Ever Life.

At the time I introduced my company, my family in Minnesota remained in crisis mode from my father's illness. I decided to create a place that would help all of us cope with the stress, but, as the company rapidly grew, we realized that many people all over the world also needed motivation and encouragement.

My parents inspired a large part of The Best Ever You Network, thanks to their positive, never-give-up attitude in spite of continuous medical setbacks. In late 2011, my dad was diagnosed with kidney cancer, which resulted in another 40-plus days spent in the ICU. During his last stay in intensive care, the nurse who was with him the most remarked that my dad was the only person she'd ever seen who could smile while on a ventilator. She said that this spoke volumes about my father.

My parents' woes actually began in 2004 with my dad's stroke, and they continue to this day. Despite the stress and heartache, however, our family smiles and does our very best to deal with life's twists and turns. Through all of this, I've learned that in those darkest moments, strength can appear if you bring it forward. You can get sucked down in the despair, or you can prevail—it's your choice. You can still be your best, bold self no matter what ails you. You have to work with what you have.

The Best Ever You Network is something I would do daily whether or not I got paid from it. It has become a way of life. One reason I enjoy this work so much is that I continue to assess what's working in my own life . . . and what's not. In the fall of each year, near my birthday, I evaluate various aspects of my life—physical, mental, and spiritual—and then I set goals and dreams within each area. I invite you to design the life you want and choose to lead for yourself. This might feel overwhelming, but try to envision your life one year, five years, ten years, and even 20 or more years out.

Let's start with what your life is currently like. What is a typical day in your life? Start with the minute you wake up until you put your head on your pillow at night. Pick the questions below that inspire you. Then take out your Percolate journal, and write down your vision for creating the Best Ever You!

Self-Evaluation: Your Vision for Your Life

Setting Goals
- What am I doing now?
- Where am I going?
- What do I want to be in the future?
- What steps am I taking to get closer to my dreams?

Attitude and Inspiration
- What is my outlook on life?
- What are my core values?
- What are my coping mechanisms? Do they work for me or against me?
- What values and attitudes do I want to embody within myself and project to others in the world?

Health

- Have I had all relevant medical checkups and exams in the past year?

- How do I manage my emotions?

- How do I cope with chronic conditions?

Money

- What has changed in my financial life during the past year?

- Does my budget accurately reflect my means and my priorities?

- Do I have the insurance I need?

- Can I make a plan to pay off debt or at least move it to a lower-interest account?

- If I've done well, what have I done to solidify my financial position?

Exercise

- How can I incorporate a healthy amount of exercise into my schedule?

- Do I need to meet with a doctor to start an exercise plan or a trainer to tune up my workouts?

- How do I manage stress?

- Can I find healthier ways to handle stress?

Appearance

- How do I care for my appearance?

- What do my looks say about me?

- What do I want my appearance to say?

- What do I like about my face and body?

- Is the time and energy I spend on my appearance appropriate to my life at the moment?

Home

- What are my goals for where I want to live this year? Am I content in my home and neighborhood?

- Do I want to find a better or more suitable home or make changes to my current one?

- Do I feel "at home" where I live? If not, what would it take to get me to feel that way?

Relationships

- How is my relationship with myself?

- Do I have a healthy balance of relationships in my life with my partner, friends, children, siblings, parents, and others?

- What is one change I would like to make in the way I relate to others?

Work
- What type of work would I like to do?
- What has changed about my work life?
- What am I doing to deal with those changes?
- What am I doing to move closer to my career goals?

Leisure
- What do I do for fun?
- Do I have enough fun or too much fun?
- What relaxes and renews me?
- What excites and enlivens me?
- How can I find more leisure time in my schedule?

Religion/Spirituality
- What is my relationship with the Divine or with the human spirit?

- What beliefs guide my life?

- Am I closer or further from my spiritual center than I was a year ago?

- Do I have people in my life who share my spiritual outlook or who can offer guidance in this area?

- Do I experience a sense of community or lack of it?

Food and Nutrition

- What is my relationship with food?

- Do I allow myself to eat something delicious but unhealthy once in a while?

- Do I stay connected to my feelings of hunger and fullness?

- Do I deny myself food when others are eating?

- Does food run my life?

Volunteering

- What do I do to help others?

- What would I like to do to help others?

- Do I readily volunteer to help or wait until someone asks?

The Long Run

- Have I made legal arrangements for what would happen to my kids if I became disabled or died?

- Do I have life insurance?

- What is my financial plan for retirement and old age?

- Have I created a living will, health-care proxy, or power of attorney?

- Have I discussed end-of life plans with others?

List five accomplishments from this year:

1. _____

2. _____

3. _____

4. _____

5. _____

Think about the future, and complete the following sentences:

- *This year, I will . . .*

- *In five years, I will . . .*

- *In ten years, I will . . .*

Percolate.
Be realistic.

Stuck in Hamster Mode

Now that you've made up your mind to start percolating and we've talked about an aardvark and a platypus, it's time to introduce you to one more critter. My family is the proud owner of an adorable hamster named Emma. She's possibly named after a pretty young actress, but my 16-year-old son won't fess up. Anyway, she is really quite cute.

You're probably wondering what hamsters could possibly have to do with percolating. Well, as a hamster owner, one thing I've become incredibly aware of is their behavior. Like human behavior, hamsters have their own way of doing things. Have you ever seen hamsters in their cages? They sleep all day and spend all night running endlessly on a wheel that takes them where? Nowhere! They run and run and, well, you get the picture—they run! They run in a wheel in never-ending circles over and over again . . . and they never get anywhere!

Let's talk about being in *hamster mode*. Hamster mode equals being stuck. You might be stuck repeating the same behavior; or you might be stuck in a job, stuck at a certain weight, stuck in a bad marriage . . . just plain stuck! Whatever internal hamster zone you're stuck on, it's important to recognize and deal with it. My goal is to remove you from that place and get you moving in a more consistent, effective direction. My mission is to get you off that wheel to nowhere.

Step away from the wheel. Get off the wheel!

Imagine if the hamster got loose from its cage and off the wheel. What would happen?

Getting out of this mode takes courage to step away from your comfy hamster zone. Let's reflect on these important questions:

- What gives you courage to ask, "Can it get better?"

- What can you do to make your life easier?

- What can you do to make your life better or more fulfilling?

- What's your first step?

- Are you afraid or hesitant to take this first step?

- What messages in your head may tell you to be afraid?

- Can you substitute these negative messages with empowering ideas of what you can and will do?

- What holds you back from fulfilling your needs?

One of the most powerful enemies you have that can lead to your downfall is *habit*. Habitual patterns of negative thinking can hold you hostage from change.

Instead of making your usual to-do list, write an "I Can't Because" list. While this might sound like yet another tool for losing your happiness battle, it's helpful to see all of your self-defeating messages materialize on paper. After you've had a chance to reflect on this list, substitute these words of defeat with empowering statements in the present tense. For example, if you wrote, "I don't surround myself with supportive and caring people," change that defeatist message into something positive that is happing in the now. Your new statement might read: "I surround myself with supportive and caring people." See how much more powerful that is than, "I *will* surround myself with supportive and caring people"? This exercise is about empowering yourself in the present, getting past your fears, and living in the now.

Below is a list to help you on your journey to empowerment. But hold on for a minute—before you attempt to run through this list, stop and consider what I'm asking you to do. Choose one—yes, only *one*—item from the list, and do that one thing today.

My Empowerment Ideas

- Love yourself, and accept your imperfections.

- Exercise 30 to 60 minutes per day.

- Forgive someone.

- Smile and laugh.

- Clear out clutter.

- Be proud.

- Eat healthy food.

- Evaluate and reevaluate priorities.

- Recognize stress in your life, and find ways to lessen it.

- Appreciate yourself, your life, and those around you.

- Give back.

- Splurge a little.

- Laugh at yourself.

- Take a break.

- Breathe deeply and say, "I am worth it."

Have you chosen your one task? You're probably wondering about everything else on this list. Well, I encourage you to pick *one* and only *one* thing per day or week. Don't rush this list! After all, change takes time. And to be honest, the items on this list can't be accomplished in five or ten minutes. Don't rush them. It should take you at least several weeks to complete all of the activities on your list. Reflect and take the time you need.

Hamsters, humans—we all get stuck in a way of doing things. Percolating helps us all to slow down the ever-spinning wheel and get off of it.

Percolate.
Be empowered.

Exactly Enough

Self-doubt may creep in now that you're slowing down and asking yourself in-depth questions. Sometimes you have these moments when your ideas come together and you become excited because everything is clear and feels like you're on the right track. Other times, however, you might struggle for clarity, grow insecure, and begin comparing yourself to others. You spend precious energy perfecting something to someone else's standards, and it ends up feeling like it's never good enough.

Regardless of where you are in your own change experience, remember that it's all good! Everything that happens is an opportunity to learn a lesson. Every day we all strive for excellence and to make each day the best it can be. It's not about achieving excellence or being perfect; it's about the intention of doing so that matters. It's about being your best, living your best, and creating the best life possible for yourself.

It's important that we know who we are so that we can stay true to ourselves in each moment. It doesn't mean that we don't have to make adjustments to fit in at times, but we can make those adjustments that aren't too much of a stretch. Loving ourselves means feeling good about who we are right now, wearing whatever we're wearing and seeing ourselves as loving, capable, and creative beings. This foundation needs to be there regardless of what we put over it to show to people.

I hope you enjoy life. I encourage you to live a life of excellence and elegance. Embrace your space. Take the time to learn new things and ideas, but overall, smile, laugh, and enjoy the journey. It's yours. *You* are exactly enough, and the space you occupy is yours to embrace.

Feeling *enough* means that we aren't dependent on anyone for our happiness. When we achieve *enoughness,* our dreams and goals are waiting for *us* to come true rather than us waiting for them to happen. We have the tools to deal with the challenges in our lives— our frustration, anger, upsets, negativity, worry, doubt, fears—so now we need to recognize that there are no excuses. We really are *enough,* always have been and always will be. Achieving *enoughness* is a gift. Peace, happiness, health, and well-being will be revealed when we choose to accept this gift. So, what are you waiting for? Open it!

Time for Reflection

It's now time for you to reflect on your *enoughness*. Take out your Percolate journal, and ask yourself these questions in order to start feeling exactly *enough:*

- Are you embracing your space in the world? In what ways?

- Are you constantly seeking ways to improve and educate yourself? If not, what can you do to get started today?

- Are you living a life of excellence?

- Are you enjoying yourself and those around you? If not, why?

- Do you feel empowered to change what still needs to be changed? Explain.

- Are you feeling like you are enough? Describe your feelings.

Percolate.
Be enough.

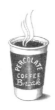

Coffee Break with Elizabeth and Dr. Katie

Shoulda, Woulda, Coulda, Didn't Change the Filter

It's Elizabeth and Dr. Katie checking in with you. At this point, you may have noticed that change can sometimes bring up old issues. In therapy, it's known as "unfinished business." It's just like old, stale coffee residue that builds up on the bottom of your coffeepot. We don't want you to dwell on the old, but instead to ask what you want and what you need. We all come with a garbage bag full of the *shouldas* we've been taught that we're supposed to want yet rarely question. *Aren't I supposed to _____?*

Many of us become unhinged when we face our day trying to do, be, and act based on someone else's rules for our lives. So let's do something radical, and give ourselves permission to challenge one of the *shoulddas* in our life.

Instead of doing the *shoulda*, be a rebel and be passionate. Better yet, desire something that you can claim without concern about what others might think. In fact, we're willing to bet that you'll find yet another aspect of your *best you* that promotes real change!

Let's think about this in more detail and reflect on the lessons we can learn from others: Imagine if Bill Gates hadn't left college? What if Steve Jobs had never worked from his garage to create Apple? What if Jim Carrey hadn't gone to Los Angeles? What if Jennifer Lopez had decided not to sing or dance? What if Coco Chanel had ignored her instincts about the fifth scent?

There are so many moments where people have trusted their intuition and have taken incredible leaps of faith to create and contribute *amazingness* to the world. (Yes, my spell-checker just did a hiccup on that word.) You don't have to be the next Bill, Steve, Jim, J.Lo, or Coco, but if you have a passion, dream, instinct, gut check, or some other realization or epiphany, don't ignore it.

Many of the people we interview on *The Best Ever You Show* have taken detours from what seemed to be the "right" thing. They quit jobs, started new businesses, and made choices that broke the rules. These decisions made all the difference. Be yourself—make your own rules, while still being respectful, of course. Dr. Katie moved all the way across the country for a better lifestyle in 2011, for example. And Elizabeth moved not once, but twice! First, she relocated halfway across the country in 1998 and then all the way across the country again for a better lifestyle in 2004.

Take a risk. Make up your own rules, and think for yourself. Be you!

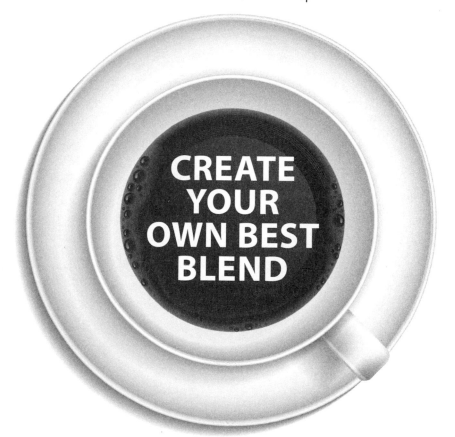

CREATE
YOUR
OWN BEST
BLEND

Switch to Decaf?

How about a switch to decaf? Just kidding! Wait, don't put the book down! I know, I know—as someone once told me, "Decaf is like white chocolate. It's fake. And it offends me." However, the idea reminds me of when I started my health kick. One of the first things my nutritionist friend told me to do was to remove or reduce chocolate from my diet. I looked at her like she was crazy. Well, I love my chocolate. I mean—I *love* my chocolate! The idea of changing to a lifestyle not filled with chocolate was something I'd never, ever considered. However, the elimination of one of my four major food groups got me to consider what could possibly motivate me do this, and this caused me to reflect on what motivates me on a daily basis. After much thought, I realized that the answer centers on my *feelings*.

I work with people to help them make life changes and live their best life. My approach is based on the idea that when you think with your heart, you will understand what you want and need to change. You will go where you place your energy. To strengthen our motivation, we have to start with our thoughts. Most of us don't change until our thoughts lead us to make better choices—regardless of how we feel. Therefore, our thoughts have to be leading our emotions to make the best choices. And—the big *and* here—some things we just aren't going to change in an instant, such as suddenly making the switch to decaf. In practice, most of us won't experience successful, enduring change until we first change our thoughts. The chatter in our mind needs to shift solidly and consistently to: "I deserve to live my best life, and all my thoughts about myself need to embrace this idea."

I think quite a lot about making resolutions at the beginning of a new year. We loudly proclaim this or that, but often by about week three, the old patterns we tried to ditch are back in motion, and the hype and enthusiasm for going to the gym has fizzled out. The thought led us to attempt to make a better choice, but what happened?

Let's think about this in reality with the experience of dragging ourselves to the gym for the first time. Just that act of kindness toward ourselves means that we have shifted our thinking. It may be as simple as, "I'm just sick of this, and I'm going to go and see if I feel better." We have to love and respect ourselves enough to give permission for us to live a better life and take a step in a new direction. Once we do that, with growing focus, consistency, and determination, we will see results. We just have to stay with it and not give up.

So let's say I challenge you to eliminate or reduce sugar from your diet for 30 days because studies show that excess sugar could be detrimental to your health. Are you going to do it? How about if your doctor informs you that you've developed diabetes? Would you make the appropriate diet and lifestyle changes then? Finally, let's say you're in the hospital recovering from a stroke due to complications from diabetes. Now will you make changes?

The bottom line is: *What inspires and motivates you?*

Does it take a full-blown health crisis to finally get you moving in the right direction? Or is it the love you have for yourself that halts a hazardous habit? Sometimes it's easy to say you're making changes only to discover that within a week of trying, you're back in full sugar mode. Let's face it, it's incredibly easy to get off track—it's easy to get distracted. It's simple to make a mental note and forget where you wrote it. And frankly, for a lot of us, there is a little inner voice that can talk us into or out of stuff or tell us that we'll just start tomorrow. It's hard to commit to something like giving up a beloved food or drink. We've all been there through dieting. We start off with such high ambitions only to be disappointed by failure.

Welcome to the Feeling Guilty Failure Land, the home of feeling like no matter how hard you try, your efforts just fizzle out, and you end up being burned out and stuck because you don't know how to change. Let me introduce you to three words to to live by: *motivation, consistency,* and *discipline.* In order to make a genuine change, you have to have consistency and discipline because these both come from motivation. It all boils down to how much you really care about yourself.

There's a great catchphrase, "Fake it till you make it," which refers to the affirmations we all use in reminding ourselves of why we want to change in the first place. We may not yet feel what we are saying to ourselves, but eventually, our thoughts, behaviors, and feelings come together and we make changes that stick.

Start by having a conversation with yourself. Find a quiet, comfy place, and talk to yourself about the importance of making small changes. Doing so provides you with the footwork to make bigger changes in your life as they appear.

Conversation with Yourself

Make a commitment to implement some positive changes in your life. Sit in silence, and think about your answers to the following questions:

- What is your commitment to yourself?

- What is your key motivation?

- Will making this change help you have a better life? Do you believe that you deserve it?

I asked you to sit in silence in order to give you an opportunity to sort out what is most important to you. Doing this helps you become consistent and disciplined, and allows you to maintain focus on why you want change so that it can be in the forefront of your thinking. Focus and attention leads you to success.

Without a clear, motivating vision and a commitment to consistency and discipline, you can find yourself scattered in a hundred different directions, and you can lose focus. Don't do that!

Let's use fitness as an example. Those in the toned zone don't sit around eating chips and dreaming of donning ripped abs. Are you wasting away in "un-motivationville"? You might be stuck there if you don't feel like doing something and then end up not doing it. There is a bigger vision that goes with that feeling. There is emotion that gets you beyond your current one, and it translates into a bigger vision. Is there enough motivation behind the emotion and enough emotion behind the motivation to go out there and get the drums and start playing, get out the computer and start writing, jog down the block and start losing those extra pounds?

Get inspired. Get motivated. Stop wishing for it, and start working for it.

In order to get motivated, you sometimes have to make way for new experiences. This can mean a change to a routine; habit; method; or something else, such as changing whom you're hanging out with. If you've been successful in seeking motivation, making changes, and understanding the difference, please share the details of your achievement. Take the time to mentor those who might benefit from your expertise. Don't be afraid that someone will steal your ideas or copy you. That's to be expected. After all, we're natural magpies for information. Imitation is a form of flattery.

Reach out to and assist others. You have so many gifts to share with the world. Have the confidence within you to cultivate greatness.

Percolate.
Be motivated.

Mild Blend with No Sugar, Please

One of the ways I've used the Percolate Process personally is by saying *no*. People love to please, and I'm a pleaser as much as the next person. Saying *no* is really difficult for me. In fact, many of us just flat-out overcommit and say *yes* when our heart is saying *no*. A few years ago, however, I swore that I would collapse if I helped in one more classroom, made one more cookie, or participated in one more activity that wasn't fully sanctioned by my heart.

I needed to plant a giant *no* in the land of overcommitted moms. As the mom of four boys, I know the feeling of being overcommitted and underpaid all too well. The moment of needing to stop doing this to myself hit me when I was talked into volunteering at the holiday craft fair. Now, those close to me know that while I can sew, I am very far from what anyone would ever consider as crafty. I warned everyone, but they assured me that they "just needed a body" for the fair.

So there I was, with a foreign object in hand—a glue gun. My task was to help children create a T-shirt tote bag. The woman who gave me the instructions put one together in about ten seconds flat. Armed with my college degree, I thought to myself, *Seriously, the kids are five years old, and she did that so easily. How hard could this possibly be?* Well, let me tell ya—kids were soon crying because their tote bags had come unglued. There they were—kids lined up for what seemed like miles, tears streaming down their faces, pieces of unassembled tote bag in hand. *Aha!* I had an idea: a stapler. That day marked the moment I received a lifetime banishment from school craft fairs.

I set a timer for feeling guilty when I decided that I could no longer volunteer at school in the same fashion as I had been. After years of serving on the PTA, working as a reading volunteer, volunteering as room mom, sending teacher treats, and always saying *yes* to whatever was asked of me, I decided enough was enough. I no longer wanted to live in the world of overscheduled and overworked families. It never fails that once you sign up for something, you become the go-to volunteer, and e-mails pour in with requests for classroom monitors, cupcakes for 150, help in the classroom, a weekend sleepover, and on and on.

"No, no, no, and more no!" suddenly came blurting out of me.

Learn to say *no,* and say it gracefully. *No* is a powerful boundary.

Although people might sometimes get angry or frustrated with you for saying *no,* guess what? That's their problem. Choose what helps you become more peaceful. Let's say you decide to change something in your life. I guarantee that at some point during the change someone will put up a roadblock forcing you to take a detour. Change often messes with those around you, especially when you make changes for yourself.

No! I don't want to switch to decaf—I'm not ready to do that just yet.

No! I don't want to lose 20 pounds—I'd like to lose five first.

No! I don't want to marry you—you're wonderful, but you'll be happier with the person of your dreams and me with mine.

Regardless of the scenario, *no* is sometimes the best word.

Let's just take my green-smoothie self for a moment. I recently started drinking green smoothies each morning and made a firm, vocal decision to remove sugar from my diet. On around day seven after my proclamation, my husband, Peter, continued buying our usual groceries of chocolate chips, chocolate ice cream, and other junk food until he finally noticed that I wasn't budging. That's when I started asking him if he'd like a green smoothie. I told him that they were changing my life, and I thought he might want to make the change, too.

After a month, Peter finally tried a smoothie, and then he had another one the next day. Within a few days, one of my sons asked for one. Just that one small change I made to my life has had some very promising results. Note, however, that I said *I* and have used the word *one*. I am still to this day a green-smoothie drinker in a house of "that's disgusting-land." My daily green smoothie makes my husband's and sons' noses wrinkle and often sends them sprinting out of the kitchen . . . but at least they did try it, and I'm still on track.

Stick to your decision, even if it messes with others. It's your choice.

Add <u>No</u> to Your Vocabulary

Go ahead—give *no* a positive whirl, and it becomes powerful and not so mean sounding. Give people an alternative *yes,* and then you don't come across as harsh. You'll still be helpful while taking care of yourself. Let me show you how:

> *No, thank you. I'd sure love to help you with this event, but now is not a good time. Can I support you in another way by spreading the word about the event to others? I'm sure your event will be a big success.*
>
> *I'm sorry, but I can't monitor the school dance on Friday night because we have other plans, but I'd be happy to e-mail an announcement to the parents I know.* (In other words, I need to just relax, watch TV, and chill out because my happiness and health come first, thank you very much!)

No is a probably the most uncomfortable word to learn to use, but once you do . . . *look out, world.*

What is one thing you would like to say *no* to?

Now in the reverse, sometimes it isn't quite so fun to have a *no* thrown your way. Learning to deal with *no* and/or rejection can be an art form. I have a saying:

"The worst anyone can say is no!" In other words, always ask or try without fear of receiving the word *no*. If someone does says *no* to you, it will usually provide you with an opportunity to learn something about yourself and to grow as a person. The person saying *no* will probably provide some explanation as to why they're responding like this, especially if you dare to ask. This is another moment to grow and change.

Percolate.
Be assertive.

Learning to Like Your Own Blend

Another lesson I learned while percolating is the value of believing in myself. There will always be people who discourage you if you let them. Having faith in yourself is the key to success. This often involves sidestepping naysayers and having a *do it anyway* approach. Believing in yourself can be difficult because you usually need to tune others out in order to find your own way. You have to create your own belief system and remember that things will be different from the past—and it's your right to have things your *own* way. You don't need a crown perched on your head, a prize, a pat on the back, a sash or medal, or anything like that in order to believe in yourself. It took me awhile to grasp this concept, as I led a life of ribbons and awards for gymnastics and pageantry. I respect pageants and pageant contestants, but for me, it was turning into a vehicle for seeking approval. When I realized that, those days ended.

Nobody can force you to believe in yourself. People can offer praise and tell you how great they think you are, but it all falls on deaf ears unless you actually believe in yourself. Ultimately, you have to choose what's best for you; if others choose for you, they're doing your work for you.

How many times in your life have you asked someone the question, "Does this make me look fat?" When in a dressing room trying on clothes, instead of asking that question, I now ask, "Who in the hell designed this?" or "Who in the world invented this?" and eventually it turns into, "Where's the nearest gym?"

I recently wrote an open and imaginary letter to yoga pants. It had a few choice words that I won't repeat here. I was bewildered by whom exactly they're designed for. I mean—who actually looks good in yoga pants? I know I don't look so great.

I know that my yoga pants Method of Operation is MOO: code name *fat*. I remember first buying these gems for myself as a Christmas gift. Well, let me tell you—it was the worst gift ever. After the holiday, which is my most terrible time to try on clothes, by the way, I took the plunge and squeezed into my new pants and asked my husband, "Do these make me look fat?" My husband, Peter, the smart man whom I've been married to for quite a long time, carefully answered, "Honey, you probably shouldn't go out of the house in those just yet." I ended up in tears, sitting in my closet blogging about the incident for the next few hours. Although I was upset over his response, the sobbing turned into a rather good inner chat about my self-esteem. I was suffering from a total belief-system failure, and it wasn't because of Peter's remark. Rather, it was because I already knew the answer in my heart.

I began having conversations with myself about my weight. Green smoothies became a regular habit, and the weight-loss process started. Although my yoga pants now look better on me and fit better than they did at Christmas, I still hate my butt in them no matter how thin I get, and my thighs aren't so hot either . . . but they're mine! I have no real, serious qualms about going out of the house in them either—no questions asked.

Let's percolate a little more.

I love entertaining at home. One time, nearly 20 years ago, I invited some friends over for Sunday-morning coffee, tea, and snacks. I bought the most expensive coffee I could find at the time. Want to know why? I thought it would impress my friends. Well, that was until my friend remarked, "This is going to be the most expensive pee I've ever taken." That moment has stuck with me like glue. I learned so many things in that one sentence.

Many people work their way through life trying to impress each other. When you compare yourself to others, you block gratitude. In reality, we all have the same fate. If it really matters to you, drive that fancy car or drink that expensive coffee, but do it for *you* and for no other reason. Do it because it makes you the best you can be. What are ten things you'd like to do regardless of what others may think or say? Reflect on it, and then write them down in your journal.

Percolate.
Be true.

Coffee Is the Elixir of Life

Perhaps the most important motivator in my learning how to percolate came when I realized that death is not exclusive or choosy. Death either has been or will be a part of all of our lives. So many wait until death is knocking on the door before they're faced with decisions on not only how to avoid it, but also how to get well. It's important to start thinking about wellness before we hear that ever so dreaded knock.

Wellness is a choice we make either as a way of life, or it's sometimes forced upon us in the form of an illness or disease, problem, crisis, or even death unless we learn and implement healthy practices. You have to decide to include wellness in your life. You can often make a small change in order to gain a huge rippling effect of well-being.

For several years, discovering and learning to deal and live with life-threatening food allergies made me feel like my world was crumbling. The simple things I took for granted before my allergies no longer existed. I couldn't go to parties and just mindlessly snack or simply eat what everyone else was eating at dinner. I couldn't buy groceries without carefully reading ingredient labels. I definitely didn't fully trust anyone else's cooking, and eating out was a total nightmare.

I felt mighty sorry for myself for a long while until I realized the beauty of my allergies. Yes, I just said the beauty of living with an illness. I soon developed a love for eating fresh, unprocessed foods. And as you know, I'm now a devoted green-smoothie drinker. Now, don't get me wrong, I have moments where you'll find my head in the chocolate ice-cream bucket as I recite my mantra that chocolate is very, very good for me because I buy the kind with all-natural ingredients. I also consume as little sugar as I can in my diet. I'm trying to be as healthy as possible, and yet at times, there are a few pounds here and there to lose and sometimes regain and lose again.

Wellness isn't just about physical health. It's also about mental health and choosing love.

What does *wellness* mean to you? How well are you taking care of yourself? Are you eating a healthy and varied diet? Are you treating yourself lovingly? Are you satisfied with how you feel? Are you exercising regularly? Do you sometimes step into your closet and have a cringe-factor moment because nothing fits?

Practice wellness.

It may be part of a new value system you implement for yourself. Practicing overall wellness has more components than just being able to squeeze into your jeans on any given day. Wellness is an overall way of choosing to live. It's healthier eating, a strong mind-set, regular exercise, and a way to reconnect with yourself when the internal critical and worrying voice(s) quiet down. It's being ready for the big event *now* instead of procrastinating and going on a crash diet days before. It's about practicing wellness habits that help you feel your best each day. It's a way of always being.

Let's think about those nagging ten pounds that just won't vacate your hips, or maybe you need to add ten pounds to your frame. If you don't love yourself and show yourself compassion, nothing will change. Find what inspires and motivates you to be healthy, and tweak it to fit your needs. If green smoothies sound scary and green, make them red instead. If jogging sounds like a marathon, walk instead. Find yourself and focus, because just a ten-pound weight loss has many health benefits. The commitment you make to yourself to shed excess pounds is often the beginning of more positive fitness and diet changes that will follow. If you have more than ten to lose, then it may be the start of an even greater weight loss. The most important thing is to show yourself love.

In a light, loving manner, try this next time you're in the grocery store: Grab a ten-pound bag of sugar or a couple five-pound bags of potatoes. Carry them around the perimeter of the store once, and then put them down and do your lap again. Notice the difference those ten pounds make. Added weight taxes your body and your joints. Losing ten pounds eases or wards off joint problems, foot problems, diabetes, and so many other health issues.

It's time to show yourself love, so let's begin by getting healthy. Here are some reasons why losing ten pounds is one step toward getting healthier and feeling good about yourself:

- **You can buy smaller clothes.** Ten pounds of weight loss is about one size drop in clothing. What a great excuse to go shopping. Shoes, too! Don't forget the shoes!

- **It's fun to exercise.** The time it takes to lose ten pounds will help you establish making exercise a healthy and vital part of your day. It takes 20 to 30 days to form a habit, and it takes around four to six weeks to lose ten pounds in a healthy way.

- **You'll discover a passion for healthier foods.** To lose ten pounds involves eating less, eating differently, and eating food that is healthier for you. Explore new, more nutritious choices, and make a commitment to your heart health. Try a green or red smoothie for breakfast each morning.

- **Your wallet will thank you.** Fast food be gone! Make a promise to yourself not to eat fast food for six to eight weeks. The biggest benefit will be not consuming high-fat, high-salt, and processed foods with questionable ingredients. Plus, you'll save money! Try saving the money you'd normally spend on eating out and putting it into a vacation fund.

- **Your doctor will be proud of you.**
  Just losing ten pounds can decrease
  your risk of diabetes and heart disease,
  and it lowers your blood pressure and
  other vital measurements. Smile at your
  next doctor's appointment instead of
  expecting to hear negatives—or worse,
  avoiding the visit altogether.

- **Your significant other will thank you.**
  You energy level increases with the loss of
  ten pounds. The hormones released from
  exercise are energy boosters! Plus, your
  sex life will improve.

- **Your stress levels go down.** Stress
  produces cortisol that often rears its ugly
  head in the form of belly fat, especially in
  women. Take a look at your midsection. If
  you are thick in the middle, look at your
  diet, amount of exercise, and stress level.
  Ten measly pounds can help decrease
  stress and stress hormones.

- **Quality family time is created.** Your
  family will see you making positive
  changes, and perhaps they'll be inspired

to make changes too. Soon, your entire household will be healthier.

You'll be on your way to a healthier you in no time. Small changes lead to bigger changes; and in this case, a healthier, happier lifestyle can be yours with just the loss of ten pounds. As I've mentioned, one way that I made the transition to a healthier lifestyle is by drinking green smoothies every morning for breakfast. And I know that some people automatically go "blech" when they hear the words *green smoothie,* but I assure you that my recipe will turn the blech into yum! Try it for yourself:

Elizabeth's Green Smoothie Recipe

1 pear, peeled and sliced
1 handful of spinach or kale
½ cup of water
4 ice cubes
½ cucumber, peeled and sliced

You can add avocado, banana, protein powder, and more to make this your own recipe. After you've added all of your ingredients, blend on high in your blender. Makes one serving. Enjoy!

One of the first steps I took toward wellness was making the commitment to myself to become healthy in all ways—physically, mentally, spiritually, and emotionally. I began the wellness journey by taking a serious look at what I was eating and shockingly discovered that I was consuming quite a large quantity of sugary foods. Several guest health experts that I had on my show also took a look at what I was eating and inspired me to do better.

I believe that reducing sugar in your diet is a critical step toward good health. Here are 25 ways that I reduced and eliminated sugar from my diet:

1. Drink green smoothies.

2. Limit or eliminate sugary cereals, and don't add sugar to cereal.

3. Eat fresh fruits and vegetables.

4. Become an avid food-label reader. Get to know the ingredients and healthy levels of certain ingredients. If you don't know what the ingredient is, don't eat it.

5. Eat brown rice instead of white rice.

6. Eat whole-wheat pasta instead of regular pasta.

7. Eat wheat bread or whole-grain bread instead of white bread. When possible, say no to white flour–based foods.

8. Nix the honey habit.

9. Watch how much cream and sugar you use with your coffee and tea.

10. Stop or limit your ice cream intake. Consider changing to something that's low in fat and sugar.

11. Watch your peas and carrots. They're very sugary.

12. Change from white potatoes to sweet potatoes.

13. Candy, candy, candy—no, no, and more no.

14. Dark chocolate in handfuls equals sugar. Don't kid yourself.

15. Pass on the doughnuts, muffins, and other breakfast sugar monsters.

16. Eliminate dressing on your salad, and switch to freshly squeezed lemon.

17. Oatmeal. *Just* oatmeal. Hold the raisins, sugar, maple syrup, and brown sugar.

18. Say no to processed, packaged foods.

19. Hold the cream and dairy products.

20. Say no to fruit juices, soda, and diet soda, too. Drink water or decaf tea.

21. Pancakes with fruit are better than pancakes with syrup. Not eating pancakes or waffles with white flour would be the best choice.

22. Eat spinach and kale.

23. Avoid alcohol or limit your intake.

24. Know where sugar lives and hides out. Here's a list of some of the possible code words for sugar, which may appear on a label. Generally, anything on a label ending in "ose" can usually be assumed to be sugar:

Agave nectar	Lactose
Barley malt	Maltodextrin
syrup	Malt syrup
Corn sweetener	Maltose
Corn syrup or	Maple syrup
corn syrup	Molasses
solids	Raw sugar
Dehydrated	Rice syrup
cane juice	Saccharose
Dextrin	Sorghum or
Dextrose	sorghum
Fructose	syrup
Fruit-juice	Sucrose
concentrate	Syrup
Glucose	Treacle
High-fructose	Turbinado
corn syrup	sugar
Honey	Xylose
Invert sugar	

25. Pizza with veggies is still pizza. Watch how much you eat, and try to use whole-grain crust instead of regular white-flour crust.

Keep making small changes. I promise you won't regret it!

Percolate.
Be well.

101

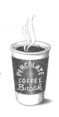

Coffee Break with Elizabeth and Dr. Katie

Sometimes You Need to Order the Boldest Blend

It's Elizabeth and Dr. Katie! We suspect that you've started to discover that one of the challenges accompanying change is encountering and dealing with those who don't want you to change. Don't be discouraged though! Instead, we just want you to learn to listen to what is said and to accept the good . . . and move on from the bad. Facing naysayers—people who are used to you being a certain way—is one of the greatest challenges when you begin to make changes. If you've always been the mom who sacrifices herself for others or the colleague who constantly volunteers to pick up the slack at the office, people tend to expect you to stay that way.

Eventually one day you may think to yourself, *I just don't want to be this way anymore.* And as a result, you start to make changes.

It could be that you come from a family of alcoholics, and you don't want to be one, too. It could be that you come from a family of over-spenders, and you're a saver. It may be that you come from a family of overeaters, and you want to choose wellness. Once you make changes, chances are that you still have to interact with the individuals who are screaming at you to go out there and spend, spend, spend or eat, eat, eat or drink, drink, drink . . . you get the idea.

Keep in mind that naysayers are those who ridicule the changes you're trying to make, they try to stop you from making those changes, and they essentially just want you to give up. They may not even realize that they're sabotaging your efforts because they're out of touch with their own struggles. They're often trying to break the cycle themselves or have yet to acknowledge their own bad habits. They aren't wrong to think the way they do, but their thoughts just don't fit yours anymore. Breaking free from their influence is necessary but can be difficult.

The best thing to do is to surround yourself with positive and affirming people who reflect the change you're becoming. Honor and respect those who knew you before the change, and make room for those who know you now. In turn, do the same for others.

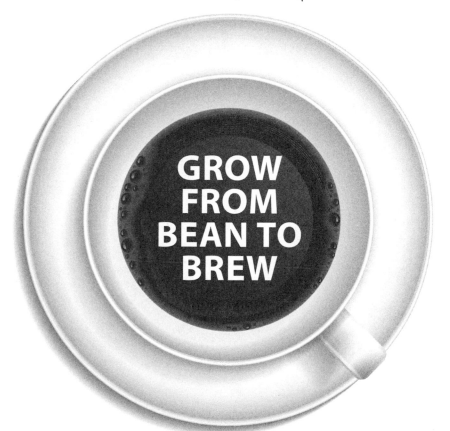

GROW
FROM
BEAN TO
BREW

Take a Small Sip

Pause, reflect, and take a small sip. Are you aware of yourself in the moment right now? I hope you're feeling empowered and that you realize the importance of each small change you can make. If you do one thing that makes you feel better, it becomes a motivator to continue and eventually becomes a habit. Selecting one thing at a time to change is an effective way to improve your life. So, take one thing—a thought, an idea, a value, or a belief—and make that a focus point. Allow yourself ten minutes each day in silence to write, think, or ponder whatever thoughts come up around this one thought or idea. It's amazing how just one small change can create the space for much bigger ones.

Here are some ideas for small changes that have big results. Please only choose *one* item at a time, even if you think you can tackle the whole list at once. When you begin, accept and acknowledge that not every day will be successful. Instead, start each day with the intention of making the change. Embrace the choices you make to follow through and forgive the times you fall short. Begin again to make today the best it can be. Change is a series of moments strung together with choices. Each one is valuable and can be made again. What is essential is that you continue to choose wisely as often as you can.

In reality, the following list contains really major changes that most people aren't able to make all at once. For example, as I've mentioned, eliminating sugar is a major adjustment. Most people will do better on some days but not so great on others. That's okay. The main idea is to do your best and make gradual changes.

Small Changes That Yield Big Results

- Drink more water.
- Reduce and/or eliminate processed sugar from your diet.

- Sit in silence for ten minutes a day.

- Write in a journal for ten minutes a day.

- Have a family dinner once a week at home.

- Exercise for at least 30 minutes a day.

- Unplug from electronics on Sundays for one month.

- Save five dollars per week, and don't touch it for one year.

- Eat a piece of fresh fruit each day.

- Say "I love you" to someone every day.

- Smile at yourself in the mirror.

- Read a book.

- Meet a new friend.

Now it's your turn. Take out your Percolate journal and create your own "Small Change Plan of Action." Here are some questions to help guide you and get you started:

- What is *one* small change you're ready to make?

- How are you going to implement that one small change?

- What big changes do you think this one small change will help yield?

Percolate.
Be focused.

Moments Matter

Are you aware of and in the present moment right now? I hope so because each moment in your life matters. You have an expiration date, and despite your wanting to claim control over life circumstances, you're not entitled to know when your expiration date will be. Life happens when you're not looking! Remaining aware that many choices don't get "do overs" is a stark reminder and can offer you courage to make choices that you might not take. The long-term effect of a moment can transform your life.

I'm not entirely sure that I agree with the idea of *not* living in the future. I think future thinking, in some forms, is very healthy as long as you stay out of anxiety and "what will happen" modes. If you change your thinking to "what *may* happen" or "what *could* happen" and think positively, future thinking can actually be fun and productive. It's like when children say they want to grow up and be a baseball player, a doctor, the President, and other occupations. That futurist pattern of paying attention to your passion, whether as a child or an adult, gives these moments meaning and purpose. For example, without carrying your love of baseball forward, you might grow to be a resentful, regretful adult who wished you'd at least tried out for a baseball team.

Your moments matter. This is why leaps of faith and risks or Gutsy Ballsy Moves (GBMs) are sometimes necessary. It's picking up the phone and asking with the greatest fear a question that could yield a "no" response—but wait, it could also be a "yes." This is when the GBM may help send you in a new direction, a new course, a new moment, a dream realized—who knows . . . all because of your willingness to believe in yourself and go for it!

It's interesting how one chance encounter, one leap of faith, or one GBM can change your life. It could be a break from your routine to introduce you to something or someone new. Dr. Katie and I have made some GBMs. I'm going to let Dr. Katie describe how both of our lives changed in a single moment:

Life changes in the time it takes to meet a person; change a thought; or, in my case, pick up a magazine.

It was 4 A.M. on a snowy day in Maine when I entered the gym, and in the time it took to put my sneakers on, I noticed a magazine called *Best Ever You* sitting on the shelf next to me. Intrigued by the title, and of course procrastinating from getting on with my workout, I began to read it. Immediately, I was struck by the simple and yet powerful message within: being your best you. The articles were relatable, not overly theoretical, and I felt eager to meet the founder of a company that for me, as a therapist, captured what I had worked years to help others understand: that simple, small steps taken in a moment can lead to lasting, positive life changes.

One workout and a phone call later, I met Elizabeth.

Because Dr. Katie made that phone call (a GBM) to me, we in turn grew to become friends and colleagues who wrote a book together. From starting the radio show to writing this book, we've made a series of GBMs and leaps of faith.

This book alone has been our lesson in being fully present while also starting somewhere to realize a goal. We've had to keep the faith; learn how to use commas properly; remove extra apostrophes and exclamation marks; and endure the drama that goes with really believing in our innocent, enthusiastic, and joyful inner-kid voice that insists on using crayons when the moments scream for them. It's about never, ever giving up.

Dr. Katie knows how incredibly frustrated I've been during the writing process at times, but writing a book is something that I *really* wanted to do. The original title and contents of this book were inspired by a sketch I drew in my journal and some journal entries I wrote called "Percolate: The ABCs of Life." With every ounce of energy I had, I turned my writings into a book titled *The ABCs of Life*. To do that, I sketched with crayons (for real) and wrote with markers, cut out pictures from magazines, and really tapped into my youth. My goal was to show how I've overcome obstacles in my life, along with other people's experiences about overcoming their own challenges. Most of all, I wanted to stress the importance of living in the moment and tapping into the power of "us and we" through the Percolate Points.

Thinking that I had hopefully written the next bestseller, I e-mailed the manuscript and the original crayon-sketched cover to seven friends for feedback: Lisa Tener, Deb Scott, Gabe Berman, Michelle Phillips, Gary Kobat, Dr. David Fraser, and Dr. Katie. And after a few days, my friends' responses filtered through:

Lisa's response: "How tied are you to the whole ABCs thing? We need to somewhat start over and get you connected to your muse."

Deb's response: "You lost me in the middle of the book."

Gabe's response: "No man is ever going to pick up this book with that title and cover."

Michelle's response: "This belongs with Hay House. You should meet [the president and CEO] Reid Tracy."

Gary's response: "Well, I'd start by gracefully romancing, perhaps deleting in some cases, and adding a little love to the expletives. Keep them inspired and intrigued even when the story is truthfully painful."

David's response: "I'm flying from Scotland to Maine to help you." And he did.

Dr. Katie's response: "I'm e-mailing Reid Tracy about this book. I've known since the moment we met that you belonged in the Hay House family. Reid needs to know about this book."

And so here we all are. With great faith, much humor, endless smiles combined with countless edits, a few new packages of crayons, the plural of platypus solidly unknown despite much research, one new hamster in my house named Emma, and a few e-mails into Betty White's mailbox, *Percolate* was published by Hay House and is now in your hands. But it all began with that one moment . . . that one phone call from Dr. Katie.

My main point is this: Don't underestimate these moments because it's amazing how much they truly do matter. Every day you wake up with the opportunity to think, behave, and relate differently; and that moment of choice is what *Percolate* is all about.

Percolate.
Be present.

The Queen of Percolate Typoland

Here's a little more about me that you should know. I sometimes struggle with perfection. Yes, like you, I'm afraid at times to try something new and have had to learn not to try to be perfect. If I must declare, I'm the Queen of Percolate Typoland.

It's something that nearly everyone can relate to: making mistakes; failing; and pressing on, typing on, and learning. Despite my college degree, I'm royalty in the realm of Typoland......!!

Oops, I just put in too many periods and exclamation points their.

Oops, I just spelled *there* wrong!

Is it your or you're? Is it there or their or they're?
OMG~~~~~ ###!!!&&& and a few --------

The funny thing is that as I just typed all of the above, nobody has crashed my Typoland gates or come to banish me to the dungeon deep within the Palace of Grammar standing so proudly in Typoland. I'm still sort of shackled to my computer writing, but with plenty of mispelings and tiepos.

Despite any amount of percolating and being enough, we must acknowledge that life is still full of typos or missteps, and that's okay; it's part of the process. I can't tell you in writing this book how many of my ….'s, !!!!!!!!, and whatever else had to be changed or removed. The entire book was even restructured.

I believe that my editors have lost some hair or sleep on just this chapter alone, not to mention the book as a whole. But one of the reasons this book exists is because I chose to ignore my inner English teacher telling me how much I had wrong and kept on writing. (By the way, if someone could insert a paragraph indent now, that would be a good thing.)

It's so easy to think that we have to be absolutely perfect before we share something we've created. I had to push past those critical voices inside of me and just write in my own style and without fear of what anyone else would think of me for making those dreadful mistakes. I write with my head and my heart, and sometimes that includes a lot of typos.

I soon realized that, still with fires blazing around me, no Grammar Guardian Knights have hauled me away for my transgressions. I have not been sacrificed to the Dictionary Dragons or drawn and quartered for my many intentional or unintentional mistakes in this chapter, or better yet for the process of writing the book. Now don't get me wrong: a few people are missing even more hair as I prolong this chapter to make my point, but I'm hear (here) too (to) tell you that everyone makes mistakes and you shouldn't let that hold you back.

I thank my editors because without them, you wouldn't be reading this. Like everyone else, I have to get help for what I can't do myself. It's that Percolate Process of collaboration kicking into full swing. There are some great editors out there, and now would be a fine time, as we go to the next chapter, for them to come back.

Oh and by the way, I initially wrote this chapter with a purple crayon on a napkin because I can! It's okay not to be perfect. (Editor's note: Only attempt this if you have a very kind and understanding editor and publisher.)

And it's okay to be childish when being creative. We need to draw upon our inner kid sometimes. As adults, we often stop doing this for fear of making mistakes. I say break out the crayons, markers, scissors, glue, and whatever else helps you feel comfortable with the creative process. How many times have you stopped yourself from trying something because you were afraid you wouldn't be good enough? Do you have a book you want to write, a song to compose, an invention you want to try? Go for it! Typos, mistakes, failures, and all! The important thing is that you're trying.

Percolate.
Be passionate.

Finding a Crack in Your Favorite Coffee Mug

Aging is a great way to learn how not to be perfect. (Amen!) Everything gets old and tired, worn and faded, if used properly in life. *Your youth will most definitely fade.* Hope that it does, as the alternative is a much more wrinkled, dried-up, deadly fate. Along your journey, your coffee mug is going to get chipped or cracked. In fact, it might even break and need to be glued together. I guess the bigger questions really are:

- How are you aging?

- Do you feel like you're 60 years old, even though you're just shy of turning 40?

- Are you doing things to keep yourself youthful?

I recall the look on my husband Peter's face when he was told by one of the best orthopedic surgeons in Maine that he would need both hips replaced. The next sentence that the doctor spoke was asking when he would like to schedule surgery as he showed him the lack of cartilage in both of his hips on the x-ray. I think he also needed a jaw replacement, judging by how heavily it hit the floor. Peter was only 52 years old when he fearlessly became one of the few people in the state of Maine to have both hips replaced at the same time in one surgery. We certainly didn't know what to expect, but a positive outlook and a sense of peacefulness for whatever was about to happen paved the way. My husband was up the next day after surgery, and by the end of the week, he was using his walker to get around the baseball field with our kids.

Don't waste time worrying that you aren't young anymore. It could be that you need to realign yourself and your priorities according to your actual age. Time is precious. Do you deeply desire to feel 20 years younger again? Then do something you really, really, love to do. Your essence is love and love is youthful, and when you tap into that, when you're roller skating or taking ballet lessons again on a whim, you'll notice that—within minutes—you turn into a kid and feel so much more youthful.

My mom says that life after 60 often feels like she's dodging one health crisis after another. I always respond by reminding her how lucky she is to have reached 60 and be agile enough to dodge those challenges. Many folks at much younger ages aren't so lucky. It's no fun celebrating chips, cracks, glue, and other mending methods, but look at the bright side— you aren't broken beyond repair. After all, there's nothing that a good, solid body shaper can't fix.

We've talked about the importance of taking leaps of faith, recognizing opportunities that appear in the moment, valuing ourselves enough to make choices that matter, and aging gracefully, but we haven't discussed self-confidence. Where does self-confidence play a part in all this?

In my work, I encounter a diverse group of personalities: people who seem really full of themselves as well as those who are extremely shy. Such differences cause me to ask why individuals are so varied when it comes to self-confidence.

As I age, I find that I'm also plagued with moments of feeling inadequate and lacking confidence. Age sometimes chisels away at your confidence. Wrinkles appear, bustlines lower, thighs bubble, and body parts hurt. When you're younger, there is a different type of deterioration of your self-confidence. It may be from a rejection or many rejections, or maybe it's someone's comment about you that lingers in your head, leaving you feeling awkward or embarrassed.

We've all had experiences like these, and there is only one thing that gets us through them: love for ourselves and from others. Even when our skirt bunches up as we walk through a crowded room, we're unaware that our nylons have fallen to our knees at an expensive fund-raiser, or that we're the only ones in costume at a party, we have to love ourselves in spite of ourselves.

Self-esteem, ego, and self-confidence go round and round fighting it out for your attention daily. Does low self-esteem affect your behavior? Does your behavior correspond more to your ego? Does your behavior match your self-confidence levels? These are constantly shifting based on your life experiences, personality, and just overall being.

Have you ever wondered whether anyone knows if you're wearing a girdle? Pardon the old-fashioned term, but anything you put on your body with the intent of shoving everything together under a dress basically qualifies as a girdle in my world. Seriously, I've had times, especially after giving birth, when I've needed to attend an event, such as a baptism, and my husband has had to help me get into my girdle. Embarrassing? I don't know. Is it actually more loving than embarrassing? He might have gently asked why I didn't buy a bigger dress, but thankfully, those words were never uttered. So, there I was at the baptism with my self-esteem, ego, and self-confidence all duking it out as I wonder if anyone can see my girdle, baby pooch, and boobs leaking (because I also have on breast pads). And my feet hurt, too, if I remember correctly while attending to my new baby, my other child, my husband, and my family and friends.

So what if we have to wear a body shaper from our toes to our nose and can barely breathe? It's not important. What *is* important is that we show up with love and compassion. True self-confidence comes from valuing ourselves as human beings, regardless of other circumstances.

What's happening in your life with aging may be beyond just discomfort. Circumstances may be seriously affecting you and your confidence, leaving you feeling like damaged goods. It could be the bottle of booze you drank, a breakup, a divorce, a bad fight, an injury, a sickness . . . this just makes you feel unworthy and drains your confidence. It's the self-loathing speaking instead of the self-love and self-worth taking over the conversation.

Whether it's extreme circumstances, the challenges of daily living, or the fear of aging, we all carry the baggage of painful reminders of our imperfections. In relationships we often wonder if people notice our scars, receding hairlines, saggy boobs, varicose veins, and the laundry list from our internal chatter of flaws we fear others might judge us by. Instead, let's put our focus on the positives with chatter such as: "I am worthy," "I am talented," "I am wonderful," and "Too bad if I don't look so sexy in shorts, I'm still hot!"

I personally think I have some of the ugliest feet ever. In each relationship I've ever been in, I've always worried that my feet would be a deal breaker, but I eventually learned to let that go and love myself fully.

Are you really "damaged goods," or are you percolating to be your best ever you . . . good, bad, and everything in between. You are loved, and love is the answer. Remember, you are supremely and divinely awesome, even with lipstick on your teeth.

Percolate.
Be authentic.

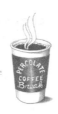

Coffee Break with Elizabeth and Dr. Katie

Mocha Moments

It's Elizabeth and Dr. Katie again! To change a behavior supposedly takes at least three weeks, and we don't know about you, but that can feel like an eternity. When Elizabeth gave up sugar, for instance, the first few weeks were brutal. Lasting change takes time, commitment, and consistency. And when life challenges us, we know that there are moments when we feel like reaching for the biggest bag of chocolate we can find and stepping into the closet to hide while devouring it. Or better yet, we pour chocolate into our coffee mugs with the hope that those calories don't count. And while we're at it, why not top it all off with a giant chocolate-chip cookie and perhaps a chocolate-milk chaser.

We affectionately refer to these situations as *Mocha Moments:* the times where you are so uncomfortable and so unaware of how uncomfortable you are that you reach for the quickest fix.

> *Wake up, and let your best self filter through!*
> *Sit still, and let yourself feel the pain. Allow*
> *the pain to percolate and inform you.*

These are pivotal percolating moments where you can find opportunities to place your energy and re-make choices of how to live and/or how to be happy with your situation. These are times when, despite curveballs, finding the positives in the depths of the most negative circumstances allows you to keep the faith and carry on. Acknowledge that you can't just snap your chocolate-covered fingers and make the pain go away. Pain has a purpose, informing you that there is something you need to pay attention to. Look at these moments as a sort of wake-up call that screams, "Pay attention!"

We hear you, and we get it—chocolate pie, chocolate ice cream, chocolate-covered cherries, chocolate cake, chocolate doughnuts, chocolate-covered raisins, and chocolate fountains always seem to be calling our name in difficult moments. When we're in pain, we re-cite a laundry list of chocolate variations, too. Trust us, we totally understand the urge to surrender to a Mocha Moment. However, we've learned from guests on our radio show who described pivotal moments when they finally put down their chocolate, turned away from the naysayers or pain, and made difficult and coura-geous choices. For instance, let's look at Elinor Stutz, the founder of SmoothSale.net, who, after a near-death experience, resolved to follow her dreams and become an author and a national speaker.

We've heard numerous examples from people who faced challenging times and made different, positive life choices. We, too, have had pivotal Mocha Moments ourselves. Sometimes we chose wisely, other times not so much, and we ended up back on the chocolate diet. But here's the thing—rather than view these poorer choices as failures, we reflected on the experiences and learned from them.

Within each challenge is an opportunity.

Recently, we were chatting about energy levels on our radio show. Elizabeth confessed that she was having a low energy/high chocolate kind of day. Her dad had been back in the ICU for over four days; and as a result, all the pain, stress, and anxiety of having a parent in the hospital became overwhelming. Preparing for a trip back to Minnesota, her suitcase was filled with bags of chocolate chips; she'd thrown some clothes in it just for fun. She couldn't snap her fingers to make it all better in an instant. Instead of facing her fears, she was diving headfirst into her chocolate safe zone.

For Dr. Katie, the hardest Mocha Moments occurred while caring for her dying mother. With each visit to her mom, a little more of their relationship disappeared while the pain grew a bit greater. Dr. Katie's drug of choice was a 20-ounce mocha coffee that she routinely grabbed at a local coffeehouse after every visit. She's now losing the mocha pounds of weight from drinking her grief away. Pain teaches us if we listen—even months later. It is extremely difficult to watch our parents age, to witness sickness, and to cope with loved ones who are in and out of the hospital. Some people appear to have learned how to show no emotion or fear and instead, show 100 percent courage, 100 percent of the time. But let's face it—this just isn't realistic for most of us.

We have tear ducts for a reason. We don't come into the world bingeing on bars of chocolate, smoking cigarettes, downing booze, and taking drugs. When babies are in need, they cry out, asking for help and seeking comfort. Adults do, too.

Let pain be pain—let it percolate, informing and presenting you with new opportunities and love. Some things clear your body of physical stress while other coping mechanisms complicate matters. Try to treat your pain with love. Reach for the tea, your coffee, the green smoothie, and make new choices . . . well, minus the chocolate.

PERCOLATE POINT #5

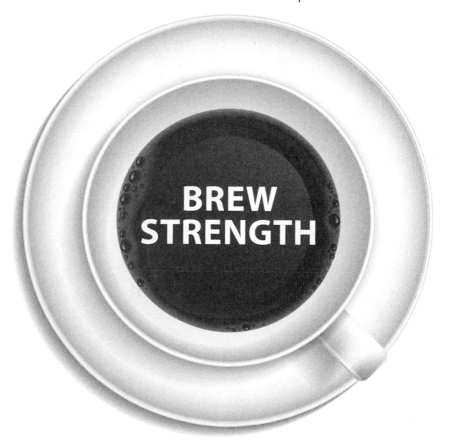

BREW
STRENGTH

A Strong Brew

Once you've gotten through your Mocha Moments, you need to take time to stop and re-percolate. Are you listening and aware when something happens that stirs excitement in you? Do you pay attention when a chance meeting with a stranger occurs? Do you ever ask yourself if there's a reason why you've met a certain person? Does the voice inside you tell you that there's a purpose or connection behind the coincidental meeting?

Paying attention to your physical reactions is an essential part of quieting your mind in order to become more aware of what's happening in the present moment. While it's important that you're out there laughing and lightening up, I'd also like to challenge you to take time to *listen* up. Take your headphones off, unplug from your devices, grab a cup of joe, and tune in.

I usually start my day before anyone in the house is awake, including the dog and cats. (The hamster is usually back asleep as well.) I sit in quiet reflection and allow some time for my thoughts to rise to my awareness.

Try to start your day by taking time to reflect in order to improve your percolating skills. Take a few minutes to think about the following questions:

- Are you aware of what's around you?

- Are you listening and paying attention to yourself and to others?

- What makes you tune in or tune out?

- Why does a fire alarm make you listen?

- What sounds like nails on a chalkboard to you?

- What sounds like the song you love the most?

- What is the sound of a person offering you money?

- What is the sound of a person collecting a bill?

- How do you feel when a person interrupts you?

- How do you feel when a person talks so much that *you* need to interrupt *them?*

- Do you ever tune out people and instead focus on the sounds around you?

- Do you sometimes go outside and just listen to the wind rustling the leaves or the birds chirping?

- Are you tuning me out yet?

Snow or shine, I often sit on my deck in our backyard and just listen or watch the birds in order to reset my listening skills. I'll bring my yoga mat out to the deck, and take a 30-minute break—from the chatter, my computer, everything—so that I can completely tune out the world and tune in to the sounds of nature.

As a radio-show host and author, I am in a profession where it would appear that all I do is talk, talk, talk. Sometimes that's true, but the key to any good relationship—whether it's with a radio guest for an hour or a spouse for eternity—is good listening and communication skills. It's all about balance. Do you practice your listening skills?

Identify How Well You Listen

Sometimes people claim to be great listeners . . . as they go on about what a good listener they are for ten minutes or longer. I always giggle when someone does this or when I catch myself doing it. There are all sorts of ways to listen. A good listener has learned to make others feel like they're the most important person in those moments when they are speaking. A good listener is aware and shows interest in what the other person has to say. However, be wary of the "good listener in disguise." This person is a people pleaser who appears to have listened to everything uttered only to agree with it all.

I want you to think about how well you listen. Take out your Percolate journal, and answer the following questions:

- Are you listening to others for messages that you may need to hear?

- Are you listening to yourself for lessons you may need to learn?

- Are you talking *to, at,* or *with* others?

- Are you off in la-la land daydreaming?

- When you listen to someone else, are you making eye contact with the person and offering your opinion or advice?

- Are you only hearing some things?

- Have you eliminated distractions when you try to listen?

- Do you take time to listen to yourself?

- Are you still enough to hear yourself and others?

Be mindful that while you might assume that someone has listened and received your message, it normally takes two to three times of hearing what's been said for people to actually process the meaning. That said, there are others who hear a message once and immediately process it, but most need to hear things a few times. For instance, instructions usually require multiple readings. An advertisement is another message that usually takes at least a dozen exposures before listeners will act upon it.

Are you a good listener, a bad listener, or somewhere in between? My hope is that you see yourself as an excellent listener. If you lack listening skills, my advice is to practice, practice, practice, and to listen, listen, listen.

Percolate.
Be quiet.

Don't Drown in Spilled Coffee

There is good that comes from every closed door or bad situation. You might have to wait to discover it—but, trust me, it's there. As I've mentioned earlier, my father has been ill since 2004. To complicate matters, he was diagnosed with kidney cancer in 2011 and had a kidney removed. He wasn't expected to live through the surgery, but he came through it perfectly. He went home, and all was well . . . until he collapsed. Medics resuscitated him twice on the way to the hospital. It was then that he began a 40-day stay in the ICU. After day two, his hemoglobin dropped dangerously low, and that's when doctors discovered that he had hemorrhaged. My dad needed another extremely life-threatening surgery to close off an artery.

None of us in my family has any idea how my dad kept surviving these critical surgeries. We think that it was his sheer will to live and our sheer will for him to survive, as we never left his side. My mom, my brothers and sisters, other family members, and I all rotated shifts so that my dad was never alone. We established this routine when our dad was ill years before. My brothers usually took the night shifts while my mom, sisters, other family members, and I stayed during the days and early evenings. It was very hard to pull my mom away during both ICU stays, but we insisted that she go home to sleep or take a break.

I will never forget one particular day shortly after my dad's surgery. All of us were looking at each other like *not this again,* dreading Dad enduring another long ICU stay and all of the ups and downs that go with it. My mom and sisters were absolutely exhausted. While I was there, one way I coped was by writing, and here's an excerpt from my blog about the experience:

> Not gonna lie. This is not easy here in the ICU in Minnesota in any way, shape, or form . . . whether patient or visitor.

Last night, after a second unsuccessful vent-removal attempt while Dad was sedated and stable, we needed a major break—and so did he. When a vent like that is removed, if the sedation wears off, the patient can be fully awake with a tube inserted down his or her throat. It can sometimes incite a riot, panic, and a constant gagging response like I've never seen before. My mom, my sisters, and I watched my dad go through this twice, only to be re-sedated and told, "We'll try again tomorrow." Watching this time was so bad that we cried—and we've seen worse than this before. Keep in mind that this is 2011, and we've been in ICU life-threatening mode with him since 2004.

I thought I could maybe cheer Mom up with retail therapy, so off we went to Kohl's. She's a fellow shoe hound like me, but she just wasn't in the mood. Shoes are like little glimmers of hope, but we needed bright stars of miracles after today, so I suggested we try the sweater department, since "Minnesnowtah" weather was calling for snow the next few days. Yes, it's colder in Minnesota than Maine! The sweaters were newly stocked and quite glorious. There we were with mounds of sweaters and ponchos purchased, but my mom still wasn't very cheery. I could tell that we both needed sleep, perhaps mounds of that instead. But rather than snooze after shopping, we headed back to the hospital for another few hours.

We decided that Dad was stable enough for us to get some sleep, so we went home for the night. We both agreed that we needed to get a little tougher for what was going to happen tomorrow: vent-removal attempt number three. Knowing the next day would be rough, I put on my new poncho and, trying to make Mom laugh, with both hands outstretched as if to fly, I landed like a superhero in her room. Then I reminded her of the line that Tom Hanks's character says in the movie *A League of Their Own*—the one about no crying in baseball. She laughed and decided that it would be our mantra for the day ahead.

We both got up the next morning at five A.M. and put on our new sweaters. I chose the poncho, and Mom put on her new long cardigan sweater. We dubbed ourselves the Caped Crusaders, ICU Warriors.

The vent was removed successfully.

Dad reached out toward my mom and immediately said, "Where's my honey? I love you, Carolyn." Those were very touching words after nearly 40 years together. We should all be so lucky. Our family is here with Dad, and he is now off the oxygen and breathing on his own.

My dad came home after some 40 days in the ICU and continued to recover. He even finished writing the book that he started working on shortly before his stroke in 2004. I'm constantly reminded of this experience as I struggle with decisions and face challenges, but just like my dad showed me, you have to walk through every closed door in order to find the new opportunities that await you. The going might get tough, but when that happens, as the saying goes, "the tough get going." Be strong and continue opening those doors. Be a warrior!

Percolate.
Be tough.

When the Coffeepot Shatters

Life is full of unalterable events. These are the unexpected, unavoidable moments that we don't plan for and never see coming. If we're lucky, most are a slight challenge or a nuisance and hopefully not catastrophic. However, regardless of the best plans and hopes, sometimes tragedy fails to avoid us.

Some occasions call on everything in your countenance to handle things in the moment and eventually learn to overcome them. Anything that shatters your sense of safety, security, and well-being can come out of nowhere and alter your life significantly. Whether you've been a victim of a crime or experienced a health

crisis, a job loss, a financial woe, a death, a natural di-
saster, or anything else that derails you, it's a reminder
that sometimes you have no control over what happens,
but you do have control of how it impacts you and af-
fects your life. These events call on your resilience and
your ability to cope and find your way through them.
Sometimes, that means making a decision to survive.

On a fall day in 2008, my brother Justin's life was
changed forever. It wasn't something that he could
have ever imagined could happen, and in fact, it's hard
for me to write about it here. I can't tell you how many
times I've typed and erased this chapter or had my parents review it for guidance.

First, let me tell you a little more about Justin. My
parents adopted him when he was an infant. His birth
mother was addicted to cocaine, so when Justin was
born, he was also addicted to it, as well as having a
variety of other health issues. In addition, my parents
learned early on that Justin had fetal alcohol syndrome.
As a result, he faced multiple challenges that he would
deal with throughout his life. Doctors even informed
my parents that Justin probably wouldn't ever talk,
read, write, or function normally. However, my mom;
my little sister, Alex, who was born nine months later;
and many in our family had a different plan in mind for
him. When they were little kids, Alex used to sit with

Justin for hours on end, teaching him to talk and didn't give up until he finally said, "Mama."

With our love and care, Justin went from a sickly baby who had little hope to a man who could talk, read, write, function at a higher level (he graduated from high school), interact socially on the computer and telephone, and make friends with people in the community. In reality, however, while excelling beyond what was ever thought possible, he was still challenged and had the social and emotional capabilities of a young teenager despite his adult age.

In 2008, Justin became a victim of a senseless, vicious crime. He was kidnapped, robbed, beaten, and burned. Thankfully, he was able to escape and despite his condition, he crawled over a quarter of a mile to a nearby highway. A truck driver spotted him and drove Justin to the police station where he was then taken to the hospital. While on the way there, the officer discovered that my brother, being a savant, knew the license-plate number of the vehicle of one of the assailants; and he could also recall the names of all of his attackers. Fortunately, Justin had survived, and all of the assailants were apprehended.

Justin went from being a happy-go-lucky young man to a victim of torture, and my family quickly learned what the term *vulnerable adult* truly meant.

Despite this unthinkable, senseless tragedy, however, Justin never gave up and was determined to survive. He gathered enough strength to crawl for help—he made a choice to live! Over time, my brother learned to cope with this event and express his feelings through poetry, and here's a sample of his work:

> *anger is anger*
> *anger makes you scream*
> *anger makes you hate*
> *anger takes control*
> *anger won't let go*
> *anger wants you to hurt*
> *anger wants you to suffer*
> *anger makes you mad*
> *anger makes you cry*
> *anger turns people against you*
> *anger is anger*

— JUSTIN CHARLES HAMILTON

What has happened in your life that you didn't foresee or plan? How did it affect you? Did you allow your own powerful reserve of resilience to help you face the situation and heal from its impact? Thankfully, most of us don't have to undergo the level of suffering that Justin endured in order to uncover our resilience, but certain events do require us to make that same choice—*to move forward.* Remember that even when the coffeepot shatters, although some things are beyond your control, over time you can learn to see the world positively once again and live.

Percolate.
Be resilient.

Help! I Need a Coffee Break

Sometimes you just need to take a coffee break. You may not be facing a life-threatening, traumatic event, but everyone has to deal with a life-altering change at some point. When the unexpected happens, some people have an uncanny ability to control the way they think about something and respond thoughtfully and calmly. The way you choose to view an event determines your ability to cope with it. Remember that it takes time to make sense of a significant loss. Eventually, one person might view a job loss as a growth experience while another person could view it as devastating. Maybe you see it as both. One person might perceive opportunity and the other—catastrophe. Neither is right or wrong, but both outlooks affect how your life changes after the event. Many people have recently lost their homes in devastating hurricanes and tornadoes; and while one person might be grieving over all they've lost, another in the same situation might be up and about, volunteering at the shelters, greeting others, and talking about rebuilding.

Many people at the pinnacle of their careers have been laid off. As a result, they often feel old, used, and rejected. Once the shock wears off, however, they may be able to view themselves as useful and very much capable and ready to seek new opportunities. They might feel power in their ability to adapt and find an even better job than the one they lost. Those who struggle to adopt a positive attitude and pursue new opportunities for growth or change could easily find themselves in a cycle of unemployment *and* depression.

So how does one rise up with a positive attitude when facing difficult circumstances? How do you put yourself in a frame of mind where you can overcome a life-altering event? How do you think your way out of financial despair? How do you find food when you have no money? Where do you sleep if you have no home? How are you going to survive without your spouse? How are you going to protect your children when you have a terminal illness? You can talk about it, but how do you really cope and get through challenges and make intelligent decisions while under incredible stress?

I can't make light of any of those issues, and I'm not going to tell you that they're all solvable with a change of attitude. However, I can tell you that whatever crumb of power you have left somewhere deep inside your soul needs to grow from being the smallest thing to a central power, or else you can never get out of that circumstance. You have to draw upon everything you have ever known as courage and find all the tidbits within yourself to put your life back together. Within you is the strength you need to make the decision that you won't let this stop you. You can read hundreds of self-help books telling you how you have to live your life, but what you really have to do in many circumstances is pretty clear. You can't wish away or change how your life unfolds, but you can control how you react and view the future.

There are also times to reach out for help. People can't help you if they don't know you need it. Although it can be hard to lean on others at times, think about it in the reverse. If your friends or relatives were in a difficult spot or needed assistance in some way, wouldn't you want to know? Would you judge them, or would you just help?

Former National Football League player Vernon Turner is an example of someone who didn't just wish his past would go away and hope for the best while moving forward. He took charge of it. Dr. Katie and I welcomed Vernon to *The Best Ever You Show* to talk about his autobiography, *The Next Level: A Game I Had to Play!* We learned all about how he went from being a 98-pound kid in high school to a running back in college and later becoming an NFL running back and wide receiver for the Buffalo Bills, Los Angeles Rams, Detroit Lions, and Tampa Bay Buccaneers.[1]

However, it was Vernon's personal story of triumph over his early life circumstances that really inspired us. His mother was a prostitute and drug addict. She had been gang-raped, and Vernon was born as a result of that horrific event. Faced with unimaginable pain and struggle, Vernon, with the help of a group of mentors, learned to direct his anger and pain onto the football field. He found a way to take care of and raise his four siblings and himself through his determination to make a career out of football. He didn't do it alone though— he had coaches and mentors who showed him how to keep the faith and focus on his goals.

In his book, Vernon mentions the influence of his former head coach, Fred Olivieri, who filled the role of father figure to him. "He took a special interest in me, not only as an athlete, but also as a human being. He took an interest in my family. To this day, I call him and tell him how much I appreciate what he's done for my family and me. I am so grateful for him."

Vernon wasn't afraid to "take a coffee break": assess his situation and reach out to anyone or for anything he needed. He also shared with us his great admiration for Walter "Sweetness" Payton, who was his idol, and while in college, Vernon wrote to him. Payton wrote back with detailed workout recommendations, and Vernon followed Payton's drills religiously. Eventually Vernon made it to the NFL with unfaltering determination and courage. All the while, he explained that his motivation for playing football was all about helping ensure that his four younger siblings' physical needs were met. Vernon Turner embodies the spirit of moving from a place of human survival to making a choice to thrive.

Percolate.
Be strong.

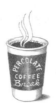

Coffee Break
with Elizabeth
and Dr. Katie

It's on the House

It's Elizabeth and Dr. Katie! When life-altering events occur, everything seems to come to a halt. Percolating stops, and, for a while, just surviving is effort enough. Justin's traumatic experience was one of those times. Elizabeth's family realized how important it was to simply love each other through it.

During these shattering events, bits of hope strung together can save our lives. Choices we make in the moment to keep on eating, sleeping, and getting out of bed every morning eventually leads to hours and even days of working through the experience. With

inner strength and resilience—and a lot of love, support, and coffee breaks—we can overcome anything
that life hands us.

Healing is a process that takes time, and when
we're able to once again percolate, it's all about keeping the pieces of hope building. One positive thought
combined with helpful behavior leads to another. Our
attitude dictating our thoughts and motivating our behavior eventually leads to healing.

PERCOLATE POINT #6

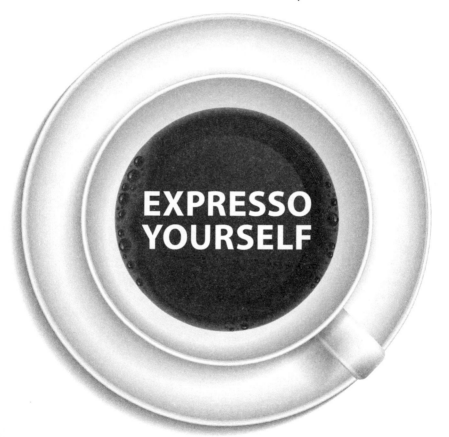

EXPRESSO YOURSELF

A Shot of Espresso

Like Vernon Turner, I've lived more than 40 years and experienced change over and over, sometimes by choice, and others because of traumatic events. I have also interviewed many people on *The Best Ever You Show* who, at pivotal points in their lives, have made choices to percolate and make drastic changes in their careers, personal lives, and lifestyles.

A recurring theme heard in my guests' stories is the importance of discovering and creating a value system. This can be tricky as we age because the values that we were raised with may not be the ones that we grow into. Our lives and our value systems are dynamic and can change.

What values do you have that guide your "big picture" decisions? Would you be able to say that you are living today in the way in which you'd want to for the remainder of your life? What would change if someone gave you a limited life expectancy? What do you want people to remember most about you? What do you want your children to view as most important? These questions can alert you to whether or not your values are aligned with your actions and lifestyle. Reflecting on these questions can identify if your values are out of alignment and bring new awareness to what you seek to change.

Does your behavior match your values? If you, like me, value cooperation, collaboration, and community, and find yourself reacting with criticism and judgment, then you are not being true to your values. Do you respond to situations rather than react? Are you generous and understanding instead of being critical and judgmental?

We usually operate somewhere on a day-to-day continuum depending on how calm and aware we are of what our wise inner voice says. When we aren't able to hear that highest self-talk, we often neglect our self-care and turn to external calming sources. Our tendency to overindulge is usually triggered by this imbalance and not being able to hear our wise messages from within. Quiet awareness and examination of our daily circumstances and this influence on our behavior can help us regain focus on our best self.

Here are ten of my most important values that I try to behave according to:

1. Practice gratitude.

2. Learn the art of self-love and self-worth.

3. Make moments matter.

4. Develop, mentor, and inspire others.

5. Maintain integrity.

6. Take responsibility for your thoughts, beliefs, and actions.

7. Live in courage, not fear.

8. Never ever, ever give up.

9. Live your life in the best way possible, and be your best ever you.

10. Embrace aging with grace, humor, and style.

What's on your list? Take out your Percolate journal, and write down your top-ten values. When you're finished, reflect on what you wrote and ask yourself if your behavior and lifestyle match your values.

Percolate.
Be principled.

Is the Pot Half Full or Half Empty?

Are you starting to move in a chosen direction toward change? In order to embrace your space in the world, you must search inward and look to the end before you even begin. We each leave our footprints wherever we go—no matter how young or old we are. You are where you are today because of where you've been in the past. Each person you've met and every experience you've endured along the way have given you an opportunity to learn, grow, and change. It's critical in this process to have faith to move forward even if you don't know exactly where you're going.

*Sometimes it becomes necessary to find
your Fairy Godmother within, and have a loving
and frank conversation with yourself.*

Have you ever met people who ask for advice and opinions from everybody and then take the suggestion that veers them off in a totally different direction? How about the person who absorbs too much information and then tries too many new things only to become confused and frustrated? Two ways we struggle to stay the course when making changes is when we constantly look to others for advice or by taking in so much information that we lose our focus. It's easy to listen to others' quick fixes, but let's face it—we'd all love to have someone offer a simple answer to our problem. The question is: Do you have the ability to not act upon advice without reflection? Not every single bit of information you come across is worth your time or energy.

There is a time and a place for feedback. However, constantly asking for advice means that you may lack self-confidence in your own thinking and choices. This can even include feedback from respected sources that might not be worthy of your energy. The Fairy Godmother is within you! Only you ultimately know what you need and what is true for you. Suggestions and supportive advice are helpful only if it fits the image of how you see yourself. I encourage you to heed the famous words from the girl with the ruby slippers in *The Wizard of Oz* when she says, "There's no place like home!" In other words, your greatest advice is closer than you think—it's within your own head and heart. You have to learn to trust your intuition by believing in yourself with self-love, self-worth, and a clear vision.

Percolate.
Be loving.

The Kind of Coffee That Never Gets Cold, Old, or Stale

I thought that a message about gratitude would be the perfect accompaniment to our thoughts from the previous chapters about being enough and having faith in ourselves. Achieving a level of inner peace through belief and trust can be a learning process. There is no question that it's very important to practice gratitude and to have or develop an opposite mind-set from entitlement. After all, we aren't guaranteed another breath, day, or moment—so being thankful for what we have truly matters.

I heard a story about a 40-year-old man who died after going out for a run on Thanksgiving. He'd had a heart attack, and I'm fairly sure he didn't set out on that run thinking it would be his last. I'm also guessing that his wife and two small children didn't watch him leave for the run and fawn all over him as if it would be the last time they'd ever see him alive. It makes you think, *Could this next moment be my last?* Now, I'm not asking you to live in fear mode, worrying about what's lurking around the corner, but rather, I encourage you to reflect on how you're living right now.

I can't help but to think of that family who just lost their husband and father. How are they going to move forward? Will they be forever angry and always asking why? What kind of attitudes will the kids have as they grow up? How will a tragedy like this affect them as adults?

It takes time to heal, and everyone grieves in his or her own way. As you journey through your struggles, ask yourself if you are more often graceful, good, and gentle or instead, if you're angry, bitter, and blaming. When things go sour, do you usually find yourself in a dark and despairing place, or do look for the grace, goodness, and gentleness that life offers, despite your setbacks?

Graceful, good, and *gentle* describe my husband to his very core. He loves sports and is an extremely gifted baseball player and golfer. He is also an accomplished and brilliant attorney. However, you'd never know any of this if you met him. He's very low-key and doesn't brag about his accomplishments. In fact, he wants his tombstone to read: *You never knew I was a lawyer, did ya?* During one of our first conversations when we first met, he used the word *kaizen,* which means "continuous improvement." That's his life philosophy. After we got married, he actually asked me if we could change our last name to Kaizen, as he just loved the idea of us getting better and better. I cherish my life with him and acknowledge what a special dad he is to our boys. His gentle, warmhearted, and loving nature is ever present and fundamental to his core. To all of us, that is precious.

Another person who exemplifies grace is Karen Fouke. I used to work with Karen in St. Paul, Minnesota. On November 3, 2005, at age 42, she was in a terrible car accident that left her paralyzed from the chest down—a total of 87 percent of her body. As a result, she became a "complete" paraplegic and is unable to walk. She remembers:

I didn't see it coming, but I recall being pro-
pelled into the air and making the attempt to
cover my head when the accident happened. Since
I didn't hit my head or suffer any head trauma, I
was conscious throughout the ordeal and can recall
many details of what happened. It's nothing short
of a miracle. My tall [5'11"] body was ejected from
the vehicle once it collided with the other car, and
I landed on my back on the highway. I was unable
to get up and couldn't move my legs. I knew immediately that I was paralyzed. It was a feeling like
no other, as a warm stillness spread into my legs. I
recall the sun shining brightly on my face and recognizing the fact that I was lying on the highway.
I prayed that I'd be safe from any oncoming cars.

The police report confirmed that a car ran a
red light going 60 mph and T-boned our Suburban
with full impact, hitting the door behind the driver.
The report stated that I was thrown 35 feet. By the
grace of God, I wasn't left with any broken bones,
head trauma, or gashes to my body aside from a
large piece of glass stuck in my hand.[1]

Karen has been featured on *The Best Ever You Show*
several times. In fact, I recently had a conversation with
her about an article I'd seen on "wearable robots" designed to help disabled people walk again. Karen responded, "I've heard about this, and I'm all over it! I've

inquired through the Courage Center and other rehab facilities in the area, and they're in the early stages of attaining these items. I've prayed for a breakthrough like this—it's such a blessing. I'll let you know when I get to walk in one!"

Now *that* is grace. Goodness is timeless. Grace is timeless. Gentleness and gratitude are timeless.

Percolate.
Be graceful.

Seeking Happiness

One of the main aspects of percolating is identifying what makes you happy. Hopefully by now, you're starting to see for yourself what brings you joy. Health and happiness are job one for most of us. *What are you doing to be happy right now?* For me, it's to smile. I'm one of those people who smiles at strangers. Often, when I see folks not smiling, I'll smile at them with the hope of brightening their day.

I believe the keys to happiness and success are being positive and leading a low-stress life, regardless of challenges and setbacks. Adjust your expectations to fit what is happening now because any improvement can increase your level of happiness. For instance, I've never been very healthy. When I was younger, coughs, croup, and ear infections plagued me regularly. I also have tremendously bad eyesight. As an adult, I suffer from food allergies and migraines. Instead of getting down, I just remind myself that my life isn't perfect—nobody ever said it would be. Everyone has challenges, health problems, or other issues, but your potential has no limit. Think about your happiness levels. Happiness and your potential are tied hand in hand like an old married couple getting their AARP magazine each month.

It doesn't take a Ph.D. in happiness to know when you're happy, sad, or somewhere in between. If you don't feel content with your life, let's work on changing that. Any chance of resolution starts with a self-assessment. So, let's get started: Are you happy? I know it's a loaded question, but give it serious reflection. You might think that the question is too broad, or maybe you just give the blanket response of "yes" or "no."

I find it interesting when people immediately nod their heads to the question. More often than not, however, their answer is really no, but they're not eager to share their true feelings. Generally, that "yes" is for the sake of appearance, or because it's really none of my business. It could also be because they've focused in on a recent trouble or situation that conjures up unpleasant thoughts. Many people often respond with: "I'd be happy if . . ." When people tell me they'd be happier if they had more money or a nicer house or a multitude of other explanations, I can't help but think it's all a disguise. No one thing or person can make you happy; happiness is a choice from within. These are merely excuses to not be happy in the present moment.

My goal is to always answer *yes* and, more important, to mean it. I mean *really* mean it! To get to that joyful place takes work. So, grab a pencil or pen, your Percolate journal, and that brain of yours; and carefully assess your overall happiness level. I'm not looking at specifics, such as, "I'm not happy because my dog just piddled on the basement floor." Instead, think about the bigger picture. Here are some areas for you to consider:

- Attitude
- Health
- Finances
- Fitness Level
- Appearance
- Living Situation
- Relationships
- Work

- Leisure Time
- Spirituality
- Your Relationship with Food
- Volunteering
- Your Overall Long-Term Vision

Does any particular category or categories stick out? If so, those areas might be longing for reflection and improvement. Ask yourself again what makes you happy, and give yourself time to really consider your answer. What could make you happier? How would you measure your happiness levels in life's "Happyometer"?

Percolate.
Be happy.

Be Robust

Taking a step forward sometimes means recognizing that you're not alone. Enduring the process of changing a behavior can sometimes feel like a grueling upward climb, but knowing that others have successfully made similar changes makes the journey a bit easier. For me, I'm inspired by people who don't give up and by those who say, "If that person can do it, then I can, too!" Seldom do I copy or try to be like someone; however, I love to pull bits and pieces from various people's ideas, although I'm careful not to draw complete pictures or visions from them entirely, as no two people are alike. I've also noticed that someone can even negatively inspire me. For instance, I might see an individual not holding the door open for an elderly person, so I hustle over to open it. When my husband and I see litter, we pick it up as opposed to walking over it. For the most part, though, grander notions and ideals inspire me.

I'm extremely inspired by men and women who *do,* as opposed to those who *talk about doing.* I find motivation from very positive people, those who have a can-do attitude and veer in the opposite direction of naysayers.

What inspires you? To get what you want, to make a large or small change, or to just complete a daily chore can be difficult at times. You might need a little or a lot of inspiration to get you going. So the question is: What motivates you when you want to quit or when you just don't feel like doing what has to be done?

Is there something or someone who inspires you? Are you someone else's inspiration? Take out your Percolate journal, and answer the following Inspiration Reflection:

- What or who inspires you?

- Where do you seek inspiration?

- How do you inspire others?

Remember that inspiration can come from personal reward, necessity, admiration, lifelong attainment, and the tenacity of the underdog. Parallel circumstances or a dream that seems impossible may allow you to mirror someone who has already achieved success.

It takes a long time to learn to listen to your gut feelings. Listen closely to see if you have any internal negative responses to a situation or a part of your life. It's when you ignore these feelings that I believe illness often occurs in various forms. Look inward, and don't let negativity fester. Be robust, and remember that you're not alone. Look to others for motivation, and try to be an inspiration to everyone in your life.

Percolate.
Be inspired.

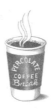

Coffee Break with Elizabeth and Dr. Katie

Self–Esteem

It's Elizabeth and Dr. Katie back for a steamy conversation. We're returning to self-esteem in order to reiterate and reinforce its importance. Small change leads to bigger change, which leads to higher self-esteem . . . and that brings us back to more change. Daily affirmations are one of the most valuable small changes we can make in the Percolate Process. Without positive self-esteem, you'll sabotage any efforts to live your best life because you won't feel like you deserve it.

What do you say to yourself when you look in the mirror? What are you thinking or how do you behave when you're in a room full of people? Are you spewing venom on yourself, decimating your self-esteem? Quick—find the antidote! Aha! It's the power of positive thinking. Inject yourself with powerful, positive language and live on. Say positive thoughts and words to yourself: *I am kind, I am loved, I am capable, I accept myself,* and *I am worthy.*

When you look in the mirror, do you criticize something about yourself? Do you find and focus on your perceived faults and flaws? Do you say any of the following?

- "Wow, I'm getting old."

- "How does so and so get her hair that way?"

- "I wish my teeth were straighter or whiter."

- "What in the world is happening to me?"

- "Things aren't where they used to be."

- "I wish my eyes were a different color."

- "So and so is smarter than me."

- "My hair looks bad."

- "I wish I had that."

- "I have a big nose."

- "I wish I were nicer."

We could go on and on with examples of negative self-chatter that we're all guilty of saying to ourselves at one point or another. The bottom line is this: Are you in love with yourself?

Dr. Katie recently attended an event where she heard Louise Hay speak about the ways in which she expresses gratitude. She described thanking everything she sees in the morning—she even thanks her closet!

One way to turn negative chatter into positive self-talk is to move your thought upside down. For example, if you look in the mirror and say, "I hate these stretch marks," you can change your inner speak to, "Thank you, tummy—stretch marks and all. You've carried four children, and I think you're amazing!" Here are a few more examples of our gratitude statements:

- *Thank you, thighs! You are/were really great at gymnastics, tap dancing, and ballet.*

- *Thank you, eyes with contacts! I can see.*

- *Thank you, smile! You light up other people's day.*

- *Thank you for my husband and children.*

- *Thank you for my health.*

- *Thank you for my family.*

- *Thank you for my home.*

- *Thank you for all of the people I will support today.*

How about you? What do you say to yourself?

We bet that if we polled *Percolate* readers and the Best Ever You audience, we would find many people who try on more than a few outfits and shoes and do their fair share of shopping for these items before an event. How many times have we asked ourselves what everyone else will look like? *What should I wear? Can I wear white after Labor Day? Does this dress or these pants make me look fat? What color should I wear?* And so on and so on!

We think about all the rules passed on from others, but we often forget about what *we* think and what makes *us* comfortable and who *we* are. It's during the times that we show ourselves to the world when we find out what we really think about ourselves. Our self-esteem is all about our thoughts and how we express those thoughts is our self-image.

What's most important is that our beliefs and our thoughts are in sync with our values. If you are a simple, nature-loving environmentalist who likes recycled jeans and a T-shirt, you won't be happy putting on a three-piece suit and having to go to a corporate job every day. If you are bright, cheerful, and socially minded, a severe black jacket may not fit your personality.

Likewise, what we say and do during our day is reflective of the beliefs we have about ourselves. Expressing gratitude means we value ourselves as worthy of receiving the blessings in our lives. If we always crave more and are never satisfied, we see ourselves as lacking and inadequate, and that keeps us stuck in a cycle of insecurity. But if we know and accept ourselves and what we value, we send a message to the world that we matter.

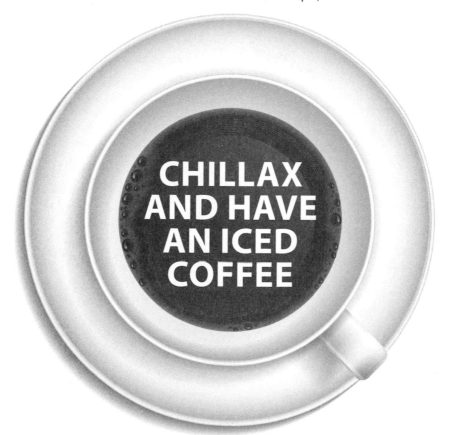

CHILLAX
AND HAVE
AN ICED
COFFEE

Laugh Until Coffee Shoots Out of Your Nose

You've worked really hard on making positive changes. Now let's take some time to enjoy life even more. Even before channeling Betty White, I tried to find humor in most everything. I am a person who can get a solid case of the giggles at any serious event and at the most inappropriate times. Since childhood, people have always at some point "shushed" me in an attempt to stop my giggling or laughter. But try as they might, they almost always end up on the giggle train with me. Trust me—this has made for some great family stories.

Let's go back there for a second and come with me to church. Picture my whole family (like all 547 of us) taking up multiple rows of pews. My grandmother Mimi is already seated because she's in the church choir and sang at an earlier service so that she could sit with the family for this one. It's the Christmas Mass, and it's now time to sing. Most of us barely utter a sound and end up doing the ol' Milli Vanilli style of faking it. We're looking up at the stained glass and are doing everything but singing the second, third, or fourth unfamiliar verses of Christmas carols like "Silent Night" and "Oh Come All Ye Faithful." Grandma not only has them all memorized, but she also sings like she's auditioning for the Met.

She really was a great singer, but she used to get so mad when we weren't singing with her. I briefly attempt a serious demeanor but then end up biting the inside of my mouth to prevent laughter. It fails, and pretty soon I'm nearly passing out on the floor from laughter. My sister Angie starts laughing, too. Before I know it, the whole row of my family is cracking up. We could count on this type of thing to happen each Christmas, and to this day, Angie and I are not allowed to sit next to each other at church. Which reminds me—ask me sometime about the Christmas when my sister, her husband, and their child performed the roles of Mary, Joseph, and Jesus.

We all have these family stories.

And did I tell you about the time I left a jokingly nasty note on my dad's car? I'd see his car parked around town, and I would put anonymous notes on his windshield. I did this for about a solid year. One weekend we all went to the movies together, but I arrived late and ended up parking next to my parents' van. I put a note on the driver's side that read: "Nice park job, a--hole!"

Now, in reality, my dad had parked just fine. So when he came out of the movie, family in tow, and read the note, he circled that van for nearly ten minutes, assessing the car's position and claiming he'd parked perfectly. During this time, he got angrier and angrier that someone would leave such an offensive note. I couldn't contain my laughter. This story, now some 20 years old, still gets great laughs from the entire family. In fact, my dad recently visited us in Maine, and we did the old, "Remember when I . . ." and my parents laughed once more.

So here's one of my favorite questions: Have you laughed at yourself today? You're looking at me a little funny, so let me repeat that: Have you laughed at yourself today? It's hard to laugh at yourself sometimes, but it could be a good starting point to add some humor into your life.

Laughing at myself is a regular practice for me. I recently appeared on TV with two mismatched shoes—one black and one burgundy. I've had toilet paper stuck on high heels, shirts on backward, and zippers not zipped. I've taken funny stumbles in parking lots while digging for keys in my purse—oh, trust me, I'm always doing something goofy and goober-like. In fact, my kids will never let me forget the time I baked a very shiny ham. None of us could figure out why a ham I'd put in the oven hours earlier wasn't cooking. My 11-year-old got so frustrated that he decided to take matters into his own hands. He opened the oven door and shouted, "Mom, the label and plastic wrapper are still on it!" All we could do was laugh. One year when we were having Thanksgiving dinner, one of the kids said, "Thank goodness Mom didn't make ham." Everyone started cracking up, and it was followed by, "You know you're loved when we tease you."

So much about life is funny or could be funny if you intended it to be. Have you laughed at yourself today?

My husband, Peter, has the great ability to laugh at himself. He's probably the world's worst drive-through customer ever. He'll pull up to the order window, and usually, a recording first plays something like: "Would you like to try our super cheesy burger special of the day?" Not realizing that it's a recording, he'll begin speaking to it. You'd think he was at an exquisite restaurant by his over-politeness to the recording when he says, "Hello, no thank you on the super cheesy burger, but what I'd like to try is the new bacon burger instead," and then he proceeds to place the whole order for the family. There is always silence. Finally, he says, "Hello, can you hear me?" and then, nearly always, also timed to perfection, the real live person will come on the intercom and ask, "Hello, may I take your order?" It is absolutely hilarious. He falls for it every time.

At one point, with four children under the age of eight, we practically lived at various chain kid-meal places. The kids would try to move to the front of the minivan to help Dad order, or they'd hide their faces while crouched in the back so that no one could see them because of how embarrassing it was. "Dad, remember that it's a recording first," became the standard cry over the years. This has become one of our favorite family jokes. It's even funnier now because he avoids the drive-through window and insists on ordering inside.

Seriously, have you laughed at yourself today?

As you know by now, Dr. Katie and I interview a lot of people for our radio program who have taken great leaps of faith with amazing courage. We know that funny and maybe not-so-funny moments will be a certainty during these interviews. We laugh a lot with our guests on the show, trying to bring their stories to a level that everyone can relate to. Laughter brings us all together.

We were recently inspired by one of our guests who had pursued a hobby at a later age. She described the power of allowing herself to try something she'd never got around to doing while in her youth. This brave woman decided to take tap-dancing classes and loved it. Whenever she felt uncomfortable or out of place and started comparing herself to others, she told us she would just laugh. I had been a tap dancer since the age of five, so I could totally relate. Having just started tap dancing again as an adult that prior year, my dancing was definitely rusty!

I decided to take my courage a step further when I learned that the same dance studio also offered adult ballet lessons. I thought ballet classes might help connect me more with my youth, as I had also been a ballet dancer. I asked Dr. Katie to come along because she used to dance when she was a child, too. Besides, it would be fun to take a ballet class together. Well, little did we know that we were stepping into a group of serious dancers who were so intense that you could feel their stares when we stepped into the dance studio.

Imagine how we felt when halfway through the class everyone had to do a series of pirouettes and grand jetés across the floor. I felt like my leaps, which sounded more like loud thumps, could be heard throughout the building like the rumblings of an earthquake.

Strengthened by our resolve to make this fun, we gathered up our best smiles and giggled our way across the floor, leaping and laughing. We didn't care what the others thought. We were doing our best while laughing at ourselves in the process. No, "grace" was not an adjective any observer would have used to describe us that first day, but they would have said that we were "fun, lighthearted, joyful, and spirited." Dr. Katie and I both continued to improve in subsequent classes, all the while keeping it quite fun.

Laugh, Love, Live: These words are plastered everywhere—bumper stickers, signs, flags . . . everywhere. Explore what these words mean to you. Did you notice that I changed the usual order? Take a leap into laughter! Lighten up.

Percolate.
Be funny.

Start Serving Up Smiles

Smiling is a part of relaxing. At the moment, I'm watching *Looney Tunes* cartoons. I really love Bugs Bunny, Daffy Duck, Taz, and the whole gang. Technically, I could be classified as a little too old to be watching cartoons, but it's my version of *Bingo Blitz*. That said, I also love to play *Words with Friends*, but I have to confess that I'm terrible at it. I figure that my shameful contributions are a good way to actually give the gift of laughter to others.

My favorite saying that I often share on Facebook or Twitter is: "Smiles are infectious; frowns are, too. Which infection do you want?"

Some people are just way too serious. Smiles never fade, and that twinkle in your eyes never fades either. Many doors open when you smile, and you may just find something you never expected.

Dr. Katie and I had the honor of interviewing Edith Namm, the author of *Change to a Positive Mindset and Extend Your Lifeline,* on *The Best Ever You Show.* Edith shared her 86 years of miles of smiles, positive-energy power, hope, health, and happiness. She also discussed how she started the Share-a-Smile Ambassadors Program, which has been adopted into several schools across the country. The mission of the program is to change the world one smile at a time by activating school, home, and community projects that help relieve emotional stress, raise self-esteem, promote positive social interaction, establish healthy relationships, and increase positive energy regardless of age, gender, or economic background.[1] That makes me smile!

What makes you smile? Take out your Percolate journal, and write down your answers. Here's my list:

- Babies
- Kittens
- Ice cream
- Bugs Bunny

- Someone else's smile

- A check in the mail

- Flowers

What makes you frown? Jot down your responses in your journal. Once again, here's my list:

- Arguing

- Bills

- House repairs

- Work issues

- Bad weather

- Wrinkles

- Health issues

Can you combine both a smile and a frown? What if your kitten sat with you the next time you paid bills? What if everything in the frown zone was approached with a gentle method of thankfulness instead of angst? Frowns generally run deeper than just the wrinkle. Frowns can be the outward sign of feeling stuck.

Let's reflect a bit more, so keep your journal handy. Ask yourself these questions to help yourself become unstuck:

- What do I do well?

- What energy, talents, skills, and personality traits help me with my day-to-day responsibilities?

- When someone asks me to accomplish a task that challenges me, what do I draw on to accomplish it?

- Am I a person who is a team player and asks for help?

- Am I an innovative thinker? Do I approach a task with self-directed creativity?

- Do I delve into a task or project with extensive research and preparation?

Make notes of the things you do well, as they'll help you with any kind of change you wish to make. Your strengths are your road map, and a smile on your face is a measure of success.

Percolate.
Be lighthearted.

Make a Plain Cup of Coffee Taste Like a Macchiato

I'm fascinated by and seem to interview a lot of athletes, particularly marathon runners. It's interesting to hear these folks talk about the joy they experience when hitting the pavement and logging the miles. I've never been able to relate to the concept of running as joyful because, well, I'm a *wogger*. This term stems from my complete and total inability to jog or run. It also reflects the frustration I feel by simply walking. I'm inspired by runners, so I combine jogging and walking and have created a new sport called *wogging*.

As reality would have it, my wogging includes some form of praying that my neighbors aren't peering out of their windows at the very moment I wog down the street. It basically goes like this: I sprint out of my driveway all dressed up in spiffy jogging clothes that have been newly purchased, thanks to being inspired again by a runner. Thinking I'm going to run ten miles, I dart from my house and then somewhere about four houses down the street, I slow down. This is followed by pure exhaustion from not pacing my jog properly, not being warmed up, and not being in shape.

So I start wogging by the time I've reached the sixth house on my street. By the eighth house, let me tell you—I've slowed to a crawl. I keep myself going with laughter, jokes, and stories. As I wog, I think about writing something funny from the experience. *Did anybody see that?* I think to myself. Then I'll console myself by thinking that it doesn't really matter if they did or didn't, so I joke to myself that I hope my neighbors in the first six houses were impressed by my sprint and that my neighbors between houses one and eight never meet to chat about my wogging. To further the joke in my head, I have to remember to sprint back past houses one through eight on my way home, and I joke that I hope they aren't all looking out their windows at the same time as they watch me cross the home finish line. If they are, they'll all think I've had a great run.

I really do find marathon runners inspiring. Wow! Have you ever gone for a mile run? Now add another—oh—another 25.2 miles! I'd like to be in better shape and be more joyful about it. While you're out there in your daily life—perhaps, wogging or walking—discover *joy*. Find a way to joyfully experience activities that challenge you.

I think it's important to remember that your joy doesn't have to be something done in order to impress people. Joy doesn't have to be a huge celebration that is centered around a specific event. Joy can be basic, but it needs to be present as you make any conscious changes in your life. For me, if something I try doesn't turn out as well as I imagined or ends up being boring, that experience very often turns into a funny blog or story I tell on our radio show.

I was introduced to joy in the form of a fitness boot-camp instructor. Even the instructor's name was Joy—I'm not kidding. With a name like that, I thought Joy would be gentle and easy on us. Well, she was until she asked me to run a mile on the first day of class. I clocked it in somewhere at around 14 minutes or so—yep, I pretty much wogged the whole mile. It was joyful the way everyone encouraged me as they ran by, trying to improve my time. I laughed when the other runners were a full lap ahead, and I could hear them close behind me. We all laughed while I improved my time over the course of the class—and that brought me even more joy.

Joy is all around. She is out there somewhere in your life.

My hope is that you become a *joyologist*. Your goal should be to spread cheer, happiness, and love to every single person you encounter. Practice the art of joyology whether you are jogging, walking, crawling, or wogging.

Remember, smiles are infectious—and frowns are, too. Which infection do you want?

If you are still breathing, you can smile. Life's an adventure, and regardless of how well you've planned it, there will always be surprises. So step, run, or wog wisely with joy and intention. Leave beautiful footprints.

Percolate
Be joyful.

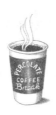

Coffee Break with Elizabeth and Dr. Katie

Filter It!

It's Elizabeth and Dr. Katie again. Before we start chatting, let's all grab a tall iced coffee . . . or how about a frappé? Kick back and get comfortable. Cool. You've learned to chill out or *chillax*. But wait—just as you began to do so, a dose of reality called *stress* hits you like a clump of coffee grinds in your mug. You just have to change your filter, and let it go. Remember what Elizabeth says: *You go where you place your energy.*

When we write the word out in different ways, watch what happens: *stress*, S-T-R-E-S-S, or STRESS! Or for those wanting a humorous approach to it, here it is backward: *sserts.* Have you noticed that you read it differently when it's written in diverse ways? It's just the way you react or respond according to what is happening in your life.

Stress means different things to each individual, and everyone deals with it differently. Although it's spelled one way, it's the impact that requires solid, bold, uppercased, and exclamation point–like attention, or else your health and quality of life can be affected.

Of course, people react to stressors in a variety of ways. For example, Elizabeth is a mom of four boys. Over the years, people have said all sorts of things to her that you couldn't possibly imagine. Here are a few recent comments: "How do you do it?" "Oh my God. Four boys?! I have two and can barely function. Wow, aren't you exhausted?" "How do you run Best Ever You, write books, do this and that, and have four boys, too?" We could go on and on. But you see, in Elizabeth's world, four boys aren't a source of stress. Of course it doesn't hurt that they're great kids, plus she has an amazingly supportive husband.

Find your own way to relax. Filter out what isn't working for you. Seek those moments when you have a chance to not only remember past events, but to also reflect on challenging situations. Read to relax. Write to relax. Remember wonderful times and dream of new memories yet to be created.

In every crowd though, there are a few type-triple-A personality critters. They're easy to spot, and you know them all too well. It's the man or woman at the baseball game or soccer match who insists on checking e-mails, texting, or talking on the phone while ignoring the child tugging on their pant leg. We've seen coaches in the outfield of a baseball game answer their phones. We've also seen parents texting during their child's dance recital. The Internet is fun—social media has certainly become a significant part of our lives—but should we be connected to it 24/7? Just think of the message we would send our children if we unplugged on a regular basis. Our kids would then not only learn how much we value them, but they'd also learn about setting boundaries, maintaining balance, and managing stress.

Be on your own quest, and ask all the questions you want to ask. Part of the journey is learning to chill out. Have you ever noticed how much easier it is for someone who is relaxed to tell someone not-so-relaxed to relax? It can be very difficult to persuade someone else to take it easy. Heck, it's probably even a challenge for you to relax yourself.

Dr. Katie uses the acronym RECREATE to help you change your relationships and manage stress. Like the Percolate Process, managing stress is about making choices every day and re-creating how you live. Every day you get to wake up and start over.

RECREATE Stress Tips

- **Rest:** Get enough sleep.

- **Exercise:** Move every day.

- **Compassion:** Help others.

- **Relax:** Make time for quiet.

- **Explore:** Try new things.

- **Affirm:** Be a positive thinker.

- **Teach:** Share your skills.

- **Enjoy:** Schedule fun activities.

By practicing these principles, you can ease the impact of stress. Like everything, stress is complex. In fact, there are good aspects of stress that inspire us to make positive changes in our lives. Stress becomes unhealthy when the activities we engage in daily challenge our ability to take care of ourselves. If we are not able to eat well, exercise, or sleep well because of what our mind considers stressful, we need to reevaluate our stressors and their level of negative effect on our overall well-being.

One thing we are learning is that excess stress damages our health. More and more research points to this: stress = inflammation = disease = shorter life. Throw in bad eating habits and lack of exercise, and you have a recipe for less than optimal health.

Now on Best Ever You, we'd like to think that we have a command on stress, a one-up if you will, but the truth is that while we talk about stress and teach healthy ways to manage it, none of us is completely without stress ourselves. You must remember to filter out the negative so that you can let it go. There are practices that we can put in place to help us ease our stress or to help us deal with it so that we return to a balanced, peaceful place instead of living in a stressed environment.

Stop, pause, be grateful for your life in its entirety, and if possible, wash away the stress with some laughter the next time you think your life has really gotten you down or you're feeling completely stressed out. When you think of the things that cause you stress, try to think of balance and relaxation. It's not good or bad; it's how you behave when you experience stress. Remember that you go wherever you place your energy. Find the answers and solutions that work for you to help you be your best self in the face of the stress monsters. Stress is a part of life, so make choices to be your Best Ever You.

We'd like you to take a few minutes to try this Relaxation Reflection. Take out your Percolate journal, and answer the following questions:

- How would your life change if you spent 30 minutes away from your computer and substituted that time for exercise?

- What else could you do with your time if you completely unplugged each night at 9 P.M.?

- What would you do with your day if your Sundays were completely unplugged?

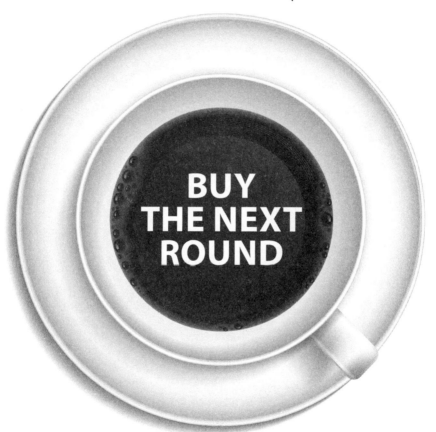

PERCOLATE POINT #8

BUY
THE NEXT
ROUND

Who's Behind You in the Coffee Line?

After all is said and done, we're in this world together, and hopefully the changes we make in ourselves will have a positive impact on others. It's easy to forget when you live your daily life that life isn't all about *you*. Instead, the world revolves around *us*. I like to do what I call the *us* check.

Let's give it a try:

- What have you done for the world lately?

- Are you showing up when you are needed?

- How often do you do something for others just because you want to—not because it's expected?

- Do you do things for others and expect nothing in return?

- Do you turn off that voice that nags at you when you can't believe you did something for someone, but they did nothing for you in return?

When was the last time you surprised someone with a cup of coffee? I love to buy the person behind me in the drive-through a cup of coffee. It always makes me smile when I see the expression of joy on people's faces when they realize that a stranger showed them kindness. What if we had days where we made it a point to surprise people with kind gestures? What a great way to move out of our own *I* place and create a better *we* and *us* space. Random acts of kindness create waves of peace.

Imagine the impact you have on another person's life when you do something unexpected. Consider the effect these actions have on your *own* life when you shift the focus from yourself to others. I think back to my parents asking our church for a wish list of needed items for low-income families in our community. I was only around ten years old, and I was shocked to see the list—toilet paper, socks, shoes, tissues, towels, and other things I just took for granted. Before this experience, I just assumed the list would include fun things like toys or clothes. It was a real eye-opener for all of us, even my parents; we hadn't expected people needing such basics. This marked the beginning of my understanding of how vital it is to give back to the community.

Although some of us might not be in the same financial position to donate, it's important to remember that giving doesn't have to have a dollar amount. Let me tell you how little things matter just as much. A few years ago, I took a bus from Portland, Maine, to Logan Airport in Boston. As I was disembarking from the bus, I thanked the driver for getting me to the terminal safely. Amazed by my gratitude, he informed me that he rarely receives thanks and said that my kindness made his day. Offering thanks didn't cost me a penny and took little effort, but the effect was enormous. We just need to stop and take the time to appreciate others. *You make a difference.* Start creating your own waves of peace and kindness today!

Percolate.
Be compassionate.

A Very Bad Brew

Sometimes being in the *we* mode means encountering someone with a really bad brew, and it can be difficult to keep a smile on your face when you get wind of it. You may even hear the potion being made: "Boil, boil, stew, and brew, this evil concoction is just for you!" Let's see, the recipe might call for a smattering of unkindness, a pinch of ego, a sprinkle of incivility, a smidge of jealousy, and a tale of woe. You get the picture!

In times when life serves you a bad brew, think of this inspiring reminder from spiritual leader Dr. Michael Bernard Beckwith: "We're all in this together. On this round planet, there are no sides."[1] Let's face it, life is packed full of people whose sole mission in life is to stir the kettle. Before you start calling them those choice words you try to only utter when no children are present or you jump to conclusions, I encourage you to pause and remind yourself that you have no idea what other people are going through. Who knows—maybe their spouse just left them, maybe their mother died, maybe they're on the verge of bankruptcy, or maybe they cut you off because they're rushing to meet a family member at the hospital. You just don't know, so give them the benefit of the doubt. You'll notice right away that you feel better when you don't take their actions or words personally. People often respond the way they do because they're reacting to what's happening in *their* lives, not *yours.*

A lot of escaping the negativity has to do with believing in yourself, your opinions, and standing firm in the face of what's bubbling on the stove and not adding your own spices to the kettle. A lot has to do with recognizing that the other person is just in a bad place, and you don't want to be in their space right now or maybe even ever. A lot has to do with your own attitude. Some people just wear cranky pants and they can't figure out how to upgrade to Sponge Bob boxers.

So mull this around a little—it ultimately falls on us to believe in ourselves, trust our own capabilities, and cheer ourselves on sort of like the Little Engine from

The Little Engine That Could. When we choose to believe in ourselves, we find the inner strength and bypass naysayers, kettle stirrers, and negative energy.

14 Ways to Be Tolerant

1. Remain positive.

2. Value your own point of view.

3. Be flexible.

4. Follow your intuition.

5. Be open to learning.

6. Don't get caught up in the moment.

7. Help find solutions.

8. Accept others' weaknesses.

9. Know your own mind and be prepared to change it.

10. Remember that we're not all the same.

11. Accept people's differences.

12. Find the humor in a situation.

13. Be compassionate.

14. Channel all energy positively.

Be openhearted and open-minded. Practice tolerance, and don't buy into negativity.

Percolate.
Be tolerant.

Best Coffee Ever!

Now that you're percolating your best brew, you have to be aware that sometimes you may want to slip back into your familiar ways and pick up that old, tasteless cup of coffee. Instead, pick up the macchiato! In order to say this is the best coffee ever, you sometimes need to *get out of your own way*. These are the words I use for dealing with situations or problems that paralyze me. Sometimes you have to get out of your own way, and perhaps, even unburden yourself, unlearn something, unbridle, and create understanding for the situation no matter what it is. Moving out of your own way is challenging because you often can't recognize that you are even *in* your own way.

The bottom line is this: You have choices. You *can* move of out of a bad situation by changing a little. Most people place so much guilt on themselves, and that's the first thing that needs to go! I know a man, for example, who accidentally hit his child with his car while backing out of the driveway. Thankfully, the child survived, but the trauma was severe for the family. It was around five years after the event that the man finally sought help after he'd placed so much burden and guilt on himself, essentially becoming paralyzed. I used some life-coaching skills to help him move forward while his therapists were also working with him. He felt like he didn't have any choices, but we led him along some new paths so that he began to feel much better as new options and ways of thinking opened up. People are often trapped in their past, and they insist on using their rearview mirror instead of looking forward. It's like being a depressed hamster on the wheel going round and round.

Talk about your past. Know your past . . . but don't live in it.

In order to let go of the past, it is important to write your life story. Write it down, accept it, and move forward. You are unique, and even if your story is filled with the most horrible hell imaginable, you'll be amazed by how either someone else had it worse than you or how your story can help somebody move on.

Think about your story. Everyone has one. You might not want to share all of the details with the general public, but everyone has a story to tell. It's the story of where you were born, where you were raised, and how you came to be the person you are today. It's a tale of twists and turns, good and bad choices, circumstance, luck, and myriad events.

The beauty and the problem with stories is that they tend to change as they are retold and shared over and over again. Facts are forgotten, details are left out, and eventually they may even become fiction. Be careful to avoid this trap.

Some say that your first three years shape who you are as a person forever. Others say that you are the person you are today because of the people you meet, the books you read, and simply from living life itself. It's probably a combination of everything. You are where you are today by living each day.

Here's a bit of my story:

I, Elizabeth Marie, was born on September 24, 1969, in Bloomington, Minnesota. I was premature and weighed just five pounds. Shortly after my birth, my parents divorced.

My mom remarried James F. Hamilton on February 14, 1975, who adopted me. When I was eight, my parents and I held an official adoption hearing in front of a judge. The adoption changed my last name, and my birth certificate from that point forward showed my name as Hamilton.

We moved to Bettendorf, Iowa, where I spent most of my childhood. When my mom remarried, I suddenly had three older sisters and one younger. My parents had more children and adopted new kids to bring us to the huge family we are today. Finding my way through this new mixed family wasn't simple in the beginning, and in many ways, it added complexities and relationships to my life that have never been easy. However, my mother and father were masters at holding us all together and presenting a united front. To this day, the greatest events are those where the entire family gets together, remembering the good old days.

What's Your Story?

Your story is your story; embrace your uniqueness and remember that no one else has the same story as you do. Now take out your Percolate journal, and reflect on your life. With pen or pencil in hand, use that brilliant brain of yours, and write down your story. Here are a few writing prompts to get you inspired:

- What are five to ten things that happened in the past that bother or nag at you?

- How have they made you better or stronger?

- What are you doing today to be your best?

We allow space for the new to begin by facing and letting go of the past. When we do this, we automatically brew our best blend.

Percolate.
Be yourself.

Reading the Coffee Beans

Over the course of owning Best Ever You, and particularly when I started, I can't even remember the number of times someone has said to me, "Why don't you just go get a job?" or "Why are you doing that?" I've also been called names and told I would never make it because I was a "washed up soccer mom" or "way too old" or—I love this one—"Who are you to tell people how to be their best?" No comments shock me anymore.

When people try to beat you down, it can be extremely difficult to stay focused on your vision and keep a positive attitude. There have been moments when

I've asked myself, my husband, and my kids, "Should I just quit?" It was often followed with, "Maybe this is all just a pipe dream, and I'm just silly and wishing for something that will never happen."

There have been two serious discussions with my husband, who at one point affectionately nicknamed me "outflow" because Best Ever You was losing money and affecting our family. Being primarily husband-funded, this was of some concern and impacted all of us. We charged forward. In fact, we moved forward with even more *Little Engine That Could* steam. There have been some serious discussions with myself about never, ever giving up and trying to refocus, stay determined, be more consistent, and even become a bit more positive.

Think of your goals and dreams as a little kid would. Go back to a moment in your life where you dreamed about doing something or had a vision of yourself achieving. Ever since kindergarten, for instance, I've wanted to write books. Since my teenage years, I've also wanted to help people overcome difficulties in their lives.

What do you want to do in this life? What is your purpose for being here?

Remember what it was like to be a child looking up at the stars? When is the last time, as an adult, you looked up at the stars and just wondered? Remember that sense you once had, when you believed in the magic of anything you could imagine really happening?

When I was three, I would tumble around the living room doing somersaults. After two years studying gymnastics, I wanted to be an Olympic gymnast. I can remember being absolutely glued to the television as Nadia Comaneci scored her perfect tens in the 1976 Summer Olympics. I did my own routines and competed—minus any Olympic medals—but that inspired me as an adult to continue my passion in some form and never lose it. I can still do handstands, flips, and cartwheels; and I marvel at the gymnasts on television. I chat with younger kids when I see they have talent lending itself to the sport and more. The passion has never left me. My family will also tell you that I'm always tapping around the house. My love for tap dancing and teaching tap dancing has never left me either.

Dr. Katie tells me that she was one of those little girls who had a deep love of horses. She was obsessed with everything horse related. Every Christmas and birthday she would run downstairs, bolt outside, and wish with all her might that a horse would be there. Growing up on a lake, there was no place for a horse, but she took riding lessons as a young teen. Finally, at age 40, she found herself living near a stable with rescued mustangs. She began leasing a horse named

Happy, and the two took long rides in the woods and along the beach. Horses remind Dr. Katie of the little girl dreamer she once was and still is to this day.

That's what visioning is all about. It's going to that part of you that forgets the boundaries, barriers, and roadblocks in your real world perspective and believes in possibility. You are only limited by your own thoughts.

Without attention to anything negative, what do you imagine your best life to be? Imagine it. Feel what it would be like to have this life. Create a vision board, or write it down in your journal. Draw it. Post photos. Get out your crayons, and don't leave out any details. Let the childlike magic flow, and allow your vision to escape!

This is the where dreams, goals, and the vision you have for yourself come into play. People may have told you once or twice to get a "real" job. Maybe you have a real job, but desperately want to run as far away from it as possible. I have no idea. Only you know what your vision is for yourself. Trust your gut, and follow your intuition.

Percolate.
Be childlike.

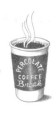

Coffee Break with Elizabeth and Dr. Katie

The Power of Our Coffee

It's Elizabeth and Dr. Katie, and we want to congratulate you! By percolating the best you, your gifts and talents can now make the greatest difference. In the previous chapters, we talked a lot about you personally, but remember that life is very much about the power of *us* and *we,* and the things we achieve together by using our individual strengths and talents. It's amazing to see what can be achieved with the power of *we.*

One person can't do it all alone!

One person sews. One cooks really well. One is a brilliant editor. One takes beautiful photos of sunrises and sunsets, and matches magical words to each. Someone is a doctor, and another is a fitness instructor. Someone just saved a life. One stays home. One teaches. One trains dogs. Our strengths and challenges go on and on and on. . . .

Your whole viewpoint changes when you discover that the world is full of people who have so much to offer if you approach them with support, positivity, and graciousness instead of fear, jealousy, and negativity. Someone's world may light up from the gift of you, your knowledge, your help, and your guidance.

Discover the people around you.
Appreciate them and learn from them.
Grow. Connect. Mentor. Teach.

One of our fondest interviews on *The Best Ever You Show* was with actress Alana Stewart, who was best friends with Farrah Fawcett. Alana came on our show to talk about Farrah's legacy; and she also told us about some of their no makeup, bathrobe wearing, heartwarming moments between two friends honestly sharing their feelings.[1]

Become someone's best asset. Looks fade, expensive jeans and shoes wear out, furniture gets stained, houses deteriorate, cars break down . . . and even you, yes, *you,* might need replacement parts at some point. In all that material stuff is the authentic you—your personality, how you treat others, and how you feel about yourself—and that's what will shine through.

Best Ever You is all about the power and potential of *we.* We share and help promote each other's ideas, and we value each other as part of a whole. Together, we create change, not only as individuals, but also worldwide, because everyone's gifts and talents are respected and valued. Our mission is to help each other be our best, and in turn, help everyone on the planet become their best selves in the process. Be an asset. Be a friend. Change the world!

◊ ◊ ◊

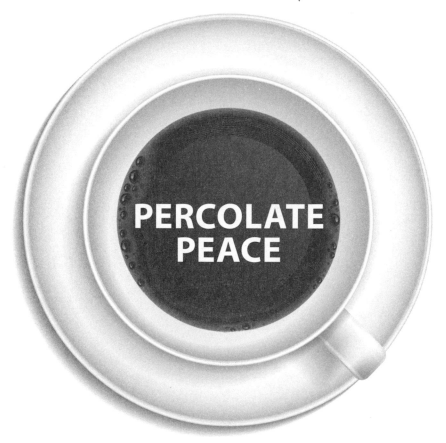

PERCOLATE POINT #9

PERCOLATE PEACE

Tap Into Your Inner Peaceometer

I felt like something was missing during the last days of writing this book. I couldn't quite put my finger on it, but I felt a need to talk *and* draw about peace. Now that you have successfully become aware of, committed to, and implemented significant changes in your life, it's time to make a difference in changing your larger world. I didn't just write this book to help individuals, but rather, to help our greatest intentions make a collective difference. If we all took the time to be our best and use our gifts and talents in service to our planet, what great changes could happen!

Now, fearing my pageant self was on a world-peace kick, and knowing that drawing is certainly *not* in my box of gifts, I couldn't quite figure out what was going on with my need to chatter about peace. With blank paper and pen in hand, I attempted to sketch something and enlisted a graphic designer to decipher my chicken scratches and turn them into something legible.

In writing this, I noticed that I got varied responses when I mentioned the word *peace* to my colleagues. Most people make fun of those who oversimplify the words *world peace*. It conjures up images of pageant contestants who have no idea how they will accomplish it and can barely point out conflict-ridden areas on a world map, yet they bravely attempt to name everything about peace that we individually and collectively desire.

While world peace starts with each of us and our understanding of what *peace* is, I really wanted to talk about the concept of *peace within us*. But even that sparked a lot of peaceful chatter about what that means. Determined to write about it, I turned inward, reflected on it, and sketched what I saw in my mind's eye. *Should I include balance? Should I include happiness? Do peace and happiness go together?*

This is my hand-drawn sketch that went to the designer.

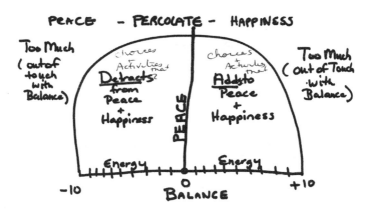

Peace evokes a placid, quiet, flowing continuum of energy and the original graphic evoked a feeling of structure and restriction. After countless cups of coffee, I finally settled on the following graphic and these thoughts to help us all percolate peace:

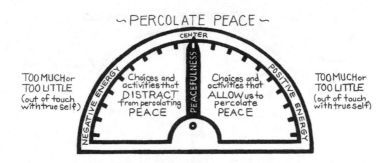

~ PERCOLATE PEACE ~

CENTER

PEACEFULNESS

TOO MUCH or TOO LITTLE (out of touch with true self)

NEGATIVE ENERGY

Choices and activities that DISTRACT from percolating PEACE

Choices and activities that ALLOW us to percolate PEACE

POSITIVE ENERGY

TOO MUCH or TOO LITTLE (out of touch with true self)

Peace is a touchy subject and means a lot of different things to people. I decided to express my thoughts while respecting the ancient origin of this powerful word and simultaneously providing a new, modern, percolated twist. I encourage everyone to be their own barista throughout this process of reflection on the word just as I did.

Wouldn't it be wonderful if all we had to do was close our eyes and we could feel peaceful? Wouldn't it be great if we just had to direct our thoughts to something positive in order to experience happiness? Peace within starts with acceptance.

You can make your lists and percolate until the cows come home, but if you can't accept yourself exactly as you are and experience that centered peacefulness, it is much more difficult to make real changes. Centered peace comes from knowing that you belong and have purpose and meaning in your life and that you exist for a reason. It's so hard to practice, though.

The goal of peacefulness or peace within is to live on the right side of the Percolating Peace graphic as much as possible. This is where positive energy, activities, and choices you make contribute to your peacefulness and positive energy.

The Heart of Peace

Peace rests within your heart. When your heart speaks, it's very important to tune in and listen. It's your own internal guidance system.

Our essence, our highest and truest energy form, comes from peace. It's still and quiet and doesn't require anything from us—just to breathe into its power. Peace is where our greatest human strength and capacity to experience happiness comes from. It's right there, and when we stop, listen, and remain awake to it, we can find our greatest source of happiness.

Peace is the key, and almost everything in life revolves around peace within.

Everything starts with peace; everything is made up of energy. The energy you bring in and put out around you and to others is light, divine, and a high vibration. When you are peaceful and happy, you connect with and to your light; you begin to percolate peace and happiness.

Imagine if you started and ended each day from peace. Are you aware of what makes you truly content? Are you thinking with your heart? Do you consider yourself peaceful and happy? How are you spending your energy?

We must remember that peace is within us. We have the capacity to teach ourselves and others how to access our quiet and peaceful selves and how to practice peaceful behaviors in each moment of our lives. We all have this ability and just need a tool or two to make peacefulness our habit.

To start, the easiest way is to breathe. By breathing, we come back to the present moment. With each breath, we get out of our head, out of our intellect, and into our body, where our heart is; and we start to feel peaceful if we allow ourselves to connect with this deepest part of who we are.

Moving fast, flying through our lives, and missing the cues that tell us we are out of balance bring us away from this peaceful place. If we don't stop, listen, observe, and experience this sense of peace because our heads are filled up with the past, the future, or checklists that block us from feeling, we miss the richness of life. Our truest sense of being our best exists here—it is our home, our now.

Peacefulness and Choices

The types of choices you make in your life either distract from your peacefulness or add to it. These choices move your energy around. Negative behavior that temporarily makes you feel good and raises your energy brings you out of touch with peacefulness. For example, addictions bring a temporary state of high, but you usually feel badly once you return to your peaceful realization of how you've hurt yourself. Likewise, you are out of touch again when you experience negative emotions for an extended period. Some people may exist being unaware of their energy shifts and unaware of their peace and happiness levels.

It's wonderful when you experience a heightened positive energy flow when you're joyful. You'll know the difference from a temporary high because there isn't a feeling of remorse but only a return to a peaceful, happy state when the joy subsides. It's the highest goal of your best self to stay there, and as you learn to percolate peace, you'll be there more often than not.

Another way people attempt to center themselves is to adjust their lifestyle by exercising more or eating right. Many people make repeated attempts, create resolutions, and put forth great effort to try to bring themselves to center. This generally doesn't work well, and usually the opposite effect occurs. In order to create significant change, usually you must find your center and then adjust your lifestyle.

In reality, lifestyle changes occur when we become aware that our ability to experience peace is challenged. To more easily return to a state of peacefulness, we begin to make small changes that eventually lead to big changes.

We would all love to stay on the happiness side of the continuum and experience constant joy, but our real life choices often require us to return to a calmer and more consistent state of peacefulness. Awareness sets in motion when we pay attention to the way something or someone makes us feel. That feeling shifts our energy to either direction.

Peacefulness and center intersect. Neither is more prominent than the other, and the energy is never stagnant. Energy is always changing, which is why it's so important to know what shifts your gauge in one direction or the other. This awareness enables you to bring your energy back to center.

What centers you?

Knowing your internal gauge or *peaceometer* is critical. When something adds to or distracts from peace, your peacefulness levels shift. One way to center yourself is to take time and remember what it was like as a child when happiness was easy to experience.

From tap dancing, to skiing, to playing video games, and more, many of us tap into the kid version of ourselves to help us remember and form that gauge of what makes us genuinely happy. Being aware and in touch with our highest self is to experience and percolate peace.

Do you make inner peace one of your life's missions? Your mission and our mission together, is to percolate peace.

Percolate
Be peaceful.

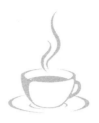

AFTERWORD

At the end of this book, I feel that it's very important to mention crayons. Yes, *crayons.* It's no secret that I'm a huge fan of them. If you were to take a quick glance at the calendar on my desk, many entries for daily activities are written in crayon. I am a 44-year-old doodle monster. (I even wrote a fair portion of this book in crayon!) It's vital for me to embrace my humor and childlike ways, and keep them with me. And believe it or not, crayons teach me not to forget my inner wisdom, my heart, and who I am at the core. I'm reminded to *think with your heart,* and *learn about and love your soul.* It's also important to do things for yourself without worry or care of what others might think.

When you embrace your inner self, you bring the wisdom, essence, and simplicity of a child to any kind of transformation.

There have been significant events in my life where I created change. These were key moments when I became determined to live my best life despite challenges and found creative ways to pursue my dreams. This is what I hope for you.

By now your old brew is no longer satisfying. It's time to order your first perco-latte. It's full of faith, grace, and *enoughness.* It's yours for the taking—reach for the latte and describe the best you.

If you could be any kind of coffee, what would you be? Remember, this is about *you.* Grab your Percolate journal and some crayons. Draw a self-portrait, and add positive words within and around your drawing that embody who you are. Tap into your inner child, and let your youthful spirit run free! When you're finished, I invite you to join the Percolate Project and upload your drawing to: www.percolatebook.com/thepercolateproject. You can also connect with me on Twitter and Instagram using these hashtags: #BestEverYou, #Percolate, #PercolatePeace, and #WWBWD.

You—your life and your moments—matter. Each day, each hour, and each moment, you have the opportunity to stop and reassess how you feel. Start over if you need to. Examine the areas of your life that you wish were different, and begin making each moment your best.

My hope is that when you get out of bed each morning and your feet hit the floor, you'll smile and be grateful not only for the coffee percolating in your kitchen, but also for every moment of every day that you're alive to experience the wonderful aroma that life is brewing all around you. Life is precious, so savor each sip.

Be vibrant. Be creative . . . and percolate!

PERCOLATE
PRINCIPLES

Be accepting.
Be assertive.
Be authentic.
Be childlike.
Be compassionate.
Be courageous.
Be creative.
Be decisive.
Be determined.
Be empowered.
Be enough.
Be focused.
Be funny.
Be graceful.
Be happy.
Be inspired.
Be joyful.
Be lighthearted.

Be loving.
Be motivated.
Be passionate.
Be peaceful.
Be positive.
Be present.
Be principled.
Be quiet.
Be realistic.
Be resilient.
Be strong.
Be tolerant.
Be tough.
Be true.
Be vibrant.
Be well.
Be yourself.

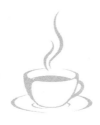

THINK WITH YOUR HEART

Apparently, hanging out in coffeehouses has brought out my inner poet. By no means would I ever describe myself as a poet, though. However, these ideas came to mind while I gazed at all of the people around me, from all walks of life. Thinking about them, I wrote the following:

*It doesn't matter if you have a jeweled crown
balanced upon your head or an old, trusty baseball cap.
It doesn't matter if you're decked out
in five-inch heels and a fancy dress, or
worn sneakers and a velour jogging suit.
It doesn't matter if you are sipping
the finest wine or the best from a box.*

PERCOLATE

It doesn't matter if the school you attend
is the highest ranked or is struggling to educate.
What matters is that you think with your
heart and strive to be your best ever you.

It doesn't matter if the car you drive is $50,000 or $2,000.
It doesn't matter if the bike you ride is $5,000 or $75.
It doesn't matter if the plane in which you
sit has placed you in the front or in the back.
It doesn't matter if the boat you buy sleeps
100 or carries just one, and you are paddling.
What matters is that you think with your
heart and strive to be your best ever you.

It doesn't matter if your job pays you $10 or $10,000,000.
It doesn't matter if your home is bought or rented.
It doesn't matter if your children have
less expensive clothing than others.
It doesn't matter if the neighbors went
on a lavish vacation, and you stayed home.
What matters is that you think with your
heart and strive to be your best ever you.

It doesn't matter if your face is smooth
and shiny or wrinkled and sagging.
It doesn't matter if you hair is full or falling out.
It doesn't matter if your makeup is on or off.

It doesn't matter if your teeth are straight or crooked.
What matters is that you think with your
heart and strive to be your best ever you.

It doesn't matter if you stand six feet tall or five feet tall.
It doesn't matter if you have blonde hair,
red hair, pink hair, green hair, or hair
that's every spectrum of the rainbow.
It doesn't matter if your jewels are real or fake.
It doesn't matter if your clothes or socks match.
What matters is that you think with your
heart and strive to be your best ever you.

It doesn't matter if you are more
successful or less successful.
It doesn't matter if you choose to stay home
and work, or choose to work in an office.
It doesn't matter what title goes next to your name.
It doesn't matter if you think or perceive
you are better or worse than anyone.
What matters is that you think with your
heart and strive to be your best ever you.

It doesn't matter what your religious beliefs or politics are.
It doesn't matter what part of the world you are from.
It doesn't matter if your skin color
differs from another or is the same.

It doesn't matter if you are male or female.
What matters is that you think with your
heart and strive to be your best ever you.

It doesn't matter if you are single or are married.
It doesn't matter if you are divorced ten times.
It doesn't matter if you are gay or
straight or somewhere in between.
It doesn't matter if you have kids or dogs
or cats or birds or fish or reptiles or mice.
What matters is that you think with your
heart and strive to be your best ever you.

It doesn't matter if you win or lose.
It doesn't matter if a medal is gold
or bronze, or there is no medal at all.
It doesn't matter if you try and succeed or try and fail.
It doesn't matter if you learn or if you unlearn.
What matters is that you think with your
heart and strive to be your best ever you.

It doesn't matter if you are sick or healthy.
It doesn't matter if you are well or injured.
It doesn't matter if you are mobile or sedentary.
It doesn't matter if you are able or if you are struggling.
What matters is that you think with your
heart and strive to be your best ever you.

Think with your heart, and uncover your authentic, best self. You'll be amazed by the positive impact you have on others. Be graceful. Be good. Be gentle, and, most important, be yourself (poet and all).

BEST EVER YOU
RESOURCES

Percolate: www.PercolateBook.com

The Best Ever You Network: www.BestEverYou.com

Food Allergy Zone: www.FoodAllergyZone.com

Motivation Marathon: www.MotivationMarathon.com

The Best Ever You Show: www.BlogTalkRadio.com/BestEverYou

Facebook: www.facebook.com/BestEverYou

Twitter: @BestEverYou

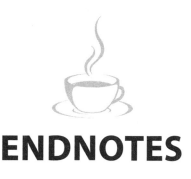

ENDNOTES

Time for a New Flavor

1. Sarah Bazey, from *The Best Ever You Show*, June 24, 2012. www.blogtalkradio.com/besteveryou/2012/06/24/sarah -bazey--mrs-minnesota-international and *The Best Ever You Show*, September 16, 2012. www.blogtalkradio.com/ besteveryou/2012/09/16/sarah-bazey--mrs-international

A Pocket Full of Change

1. Debra Oakland, from *The Best Ever You Show*, March 27, 2012. www.blogtalkradio.com/besteveryou/2012/03/27/ debra-oakland--living-in-courage

2. Brian and Kathy Hom, from *The Best Ever You Show*, September 25, 2011. www.blogtalkradio.com/besteveryou/2011/09/25/ food-allergies-brian-hom-sarah-shannon-paul-vondermeulen and *Best Ever You Magazine*, July 2011.

Help! I Need a Coffee Break

1. Vernon Turner, from *The Best Ever You Show*, November 20, 2012. www.blogtalkradio.com/besteveryou/2012/11/20/vernon-turner

The Kind of Coffee That Never Gets Cold, Old, or Stale

1. Karen Fouke, from Best Ever You, October 7, 2012.
   www.besteveryou.com

Start Serving Up Smiles

1. Edith Namm, from *The Best Ever You Show*, November 27, 2012.
   www.blogtalkradio.com/besteveryou/2012/11/27/edith-namm

A Very Bad Brew

1. Michael Bernard Beckwith, from The Motivation Marathon,
   January 2012.

Coffee Break with Elizabeth and Dr. Katie:
The Power of Our Coffee

1. Alana Stewart, from *The Best Ever You Show*, November 16, 2010.
   www.blogtalkradio.com/besteveryou/2010/11/16/
   elizabeth-and-katie-live-with-alana-stewart

ACKNOWLEDGMENTS

When you make a decision to write a book, you forever change yourself and those around you. I can look back at everything that has happened in my life and now more clearly see how and why I wrote this. I thought I had some serious typos in my life, but they were really blessings to be counted and recounted. It could take another book just to thank everyone because I believe I've met each and every person in my life for a reason.

I wish to start by thanking my husband, Peter. Without the loving support and understanding I received from him and our four boys, Connor, Quinn, Cam, and Quaid, this book would not have been possible. Thank you for your love, infinite patience, and encouragement. I love you all dearly. You each inspire me to be my very best daily.

I am eternally grateful to my mom, Carolyn Hamilton, for her moments of deep courage to remove us both from a terrible situation when we were young and point us in a different direction. Throughout my life, I've always marveled at my parents' profound love for one another, their deep courage, and their never-give-up attitudes. Never did I think they would be so challenged with the various health crises they have faced. Seeing all they have gone through has taught me to put things into greater perspective and have an even deeper understanding of what love, compassion, and "till death do us part" really mean. I love you both dearly. Thank you for all you have done in my life.

My brother Justin's resilience and love of life have always inspired me. I have an old picture of him that sits on my desk. He is five in the photo, there's paint splattered all behind him, and he has a huge smile on his face. Justin has a smile on his face almost all the time, and he's genuinely caring of others. He also has a tremendous capability to forgive when it would be so easy to remain angry. Thank you, Justin, for allowing me to share your story and your poem. I love you.

I don't always answer the phone when it rings. However, I'm grateful I did on the day that Dr. Katie Eastman decided to call me. Without Dr. Katie and her level of excellence in listening, writing, psychology, companionship, and love of shoes, this book definitely wouldn't have been possible. Thank you so much.

On our journey, we meet people who change and inspire us. Sarah Bazey, Karen Fouke, Debra Oakland, Edith Namm, Brian Hom and the Hom family, and Vernon Turner were each willing to step forward and share their incredible stories with our readers. When I asked each of them if I could include their experiences in this book, they responded within just a few short minutes and took the opportunity to continue to change the lives of others by sharing their pain and stories of hope. Thank you always.

I am so incredibly grateful to everyone at the MedicAlert Foundation for all of the support you've given me over the years. The MedicAlert Foundation has allowed me to raise awareness internationally and to help make a difference and save lives as a spokesperson since 2006 and as a member since 1998.

Thank you also to the following people who helped with this book: Sandra Waugh, for her amazing artwork; Lisa Tener, for her guidance, patience, editing, reediting, love, support, and muse idea; and Deb Scott, Liz Foley, Emily Davis Janson, and Katana Abbott for your early and continued involvement with *Percolate*.

A chance meeting with Deb Scott has forever changed my path and the crowd of people I encounter on it. It's funny; we even tossed around the idea at first of writing this book together. We didn't, but Deb has been in the background reviewing each word written and is responsible for connecting me with many of the #BestPeople who have helped bring this book to life. Deb and I have gone on to work together now for several years, collaborating on projects such as The Motivation Marathon, with millions of global listeners on our radio shows and in social media. Thank you so much, Deb. (p.s. You're right about the different directions people can take you in!)

Taking a walk in someone else's shoes can be a real eye-opener. Well, I raided Shea Vaughn's shoe closet. Not only did Shea loan me her shoes, which were way cooler than any I've ever owned, but I also discovered the best vegetable peeler that TSA somehow didn't confiscate from my luggage on my return to Maine from Chicago. It's a long story, but in short, I send a huge thank-you to Shea. She and her husband, Steve, are all heart. They opened their lives and home to my family and me, and continue to be extraordinary friends and sources of wisdom and laughter. Thank you always.

Once in a while life graces us in the most unexpected ways. For me, that graceful presence came in the form of Lynn Abbott-McCloud. Lynn has an incredible gift and energy. She took the book on as a project for her editing class at the University of North Carolina at Charlotte and has been with me every step of the way in editing this entire book. Lynn has an incredible knack for recognizing and respecting the author's voice. She helped maintain my personality throughout, while also making my sentences clearer, helping me choose interesting words, and of course, ensuring commas were where they were supposed to be. And yes, it was incredibly challenging for her to scroll through "The Queen of Percolate Typoland."

I'd like to thank actor Michael McGlone for being such a great friend and support. Along the way, I met author Gabe Berman, who has showed me how to "live like a fruit fly." Thank you for your support and encouragement in helping me write this book.

These acknowledgments wouldn't be complete without including my friend David Fraser, who has a meticulous eye for detail, incredible insight, and apparently likes to fly. He not only took a plane from Scotland to Boston to help me, but he has also placed his genuine trust and faith in this project from start to finish.

Since I was a kid, I've always known there was something special about Frank Stallone. I just love him and his music. Imagine my smile when his manager, Randi Siegel, arranged for him to be a guest on my radio show and on *Best Ever You* magazine's cover and feature story. Frank turned out to be even more graceful, elegant, and beautiful than I ever expected. And I'm not the only one who adores him. Our magazine downloads soared, and we had more listeners than ever on the radio show. People treasured our interviews with Frank. In all of that, I discovered an incredible and brilliant friend in Randi Siegel. She says she's not very funny, but note that she's the one who helped launch Jimmy Fallon's career. I learn something new, interesting, and inspirational each time I speak with Randi; and for that, I asked if she would write the Foreword for *Percolate*. So, a very special thank-you goes out to both Randi and Frank for their trust, faith, and love.

Speaking of trust, faith, and love, seldom am I left at a loss for additional words, but I find myself somewhat unable to express the magnitude of appreciation for everyone at Hay House. Thank you all for taking me under your wings and showing me how to fly. And thanks for welcoming me into your family and hugging me from over 3,000 miles away. You are all a true joy to work with, and you've helped me be my very best. Thank you!

Every so often you meet someone you feel as if you've known your whole life. The person could even be across the world, or in this case, across the country. Gary Kobat, who also loves all things cats and baseball, is one of the finest people I know. If you have just a brief moment to talk to him, he will change your life for the better.

Thank you to the emergency responders in Prior Lake, Minnesota, and the ER doctors at Fairview Ridges Hospital in Burnsville, Minnesota. I wouldn't be here without you.

Finally, I wish to give a very special thank-you to the followers and supporters of The Best Ever You Network. The Best Ever You community continues to inspire me. You are the *you* in Best Ever You . . . *you are the best!*

With love, hugs, and endless gratitude,
Elizabeth

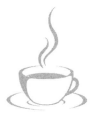

ABOUT THE AUTHORS

Elizabeth Hamilton-Guarino learned early on to live her life with purpose and meaning. Since her teenage years, she has worked to raise awareness on issues near and dear to her heart, including the prevention of drinking and driving, children's literacy, stroke and diabetes awareness, and food-allergy education and awareness. She also discovered the power of radio, television, and print, which led her into a career as a broadcaster, spokesperson, radio/television personality, and writer.

In 1998, Elizabeth nearly lost her life from an allergic reaction to almonds. Following pregnancy, she'd developed anaphylaxis to multiple foods, including nuts, peanuts, fish, and shellfish. In 1999, she suffered a second near-fatal reaction while pregnant with her third son. She and her unborn child were hospitalized for over a week in Minnesota following that reaction.

When Elizabeth met her husband, Peter, on November 7, 1998, she became inspired to refocus her message on change. Over several years, their growing family made a series of moves from the Midwest to the West Coast, and then on to the East Coast. All the while, they made a series of gradual improvements to their lives that have brought them to this point and which continue guiding them forward.

In 2006, Elizabeth became a food-allergy spokesperson for the MedicAlert Foundation (www.Medic Alert.org) and appeared in their magazine, which was mailed to over a million members. She continues her role as a spokesperson today, working closely with the foundation's executive team and appearing on their website to help raise food-allergy awareness internationally. Elizabeth is also featured in the book *One of the Gang: Nurturing the Souls of Children with Food Allergies* by Gina Clowes. In 2014, she became a spokesperson for the Food Allergy & Anaphylaxis Connection Team, FAACT (www.foodallergyawareness.org).

In 2008, Elizabeth quit a 17-year career in the financial-services industry in order to start The Best Ever You Network. She understands firsthand the challenges life can bring and has worked with people worldwide to illuminate their light within and help them uncover their best life. As the CEO and founder, guiding spirit, and energy behind the Best Ever You brand, Elizabeth loves nothing more than bringing audiences together with the encouragement and inspiration they need.

Elizabeth has a bachelor's degree, cum laude, in mass communications and broadcasting from St. Ambrose University in Davenport, Iowa. Elizabeth, Peter, and their four wonderful boys reside in Maine. You can connect with Elizabeth on Twitter and Instagram using these hashtags: #BestEverYou, #Percolate, #Percolate Peace, and #WWBWD. Learn more at www.BestEverYou .com and www.PercolateBook.com.

Dr. Katie Eastman has been a change agent from a very young age. Listening to friends who always turned to her for advice became a way of being. She was the "Dear Abby" of the fifth grade and learned to empathize with and value who and what others were trying to be.

Thus, it was natural for Dr. Katie to choose a profession where she would help people become their best selves by listening and reflecting back what they wished to become. It was even more natural to work with children, who have always been Dr. Katie's greatest teachers. Marveling at their ability to be present, joyful, and grateful in some of the most challenging circumstances, Dr. Katie (which is her nickname given to her by a child patient) shares with Elizabeth the value of bringing childlike simplicity together with complex human issues.

Dr. Katie holds a doctorate in clinical child psychology and a master's in social work, and she also did extensive study in theology. Directing these skills to work in hospice and palliative care, she has become a tireless advocate for valuing quality of life throughout an individual's life span and is the founder of Children's Palliative Care Community. Learn more about Dr. Katie and her work at www.DrKatieEastman.net.

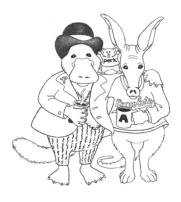

No hamsters or aardvarks were harmed in making, creating, or thinking about this book. I left the platypus alone, too. I still don't know the plural.

Oh, and by the way, my illustrator first drew an armadillo instead of an aardvark by mistake. He wasn't harmed either, although I'm still struggling with the plural there, too. *Armadilli?*

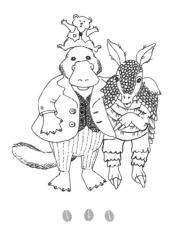

We hope you enjoyed this Hay House book. If you'd like
to receive our online catalog featuring additional information
on Hay House books and products, or if you'd like to find
out more about the Hay Foundation, please contact:

Hay House, Inc., P.O. Box 5100, Carlsbad, CA 92018-5100
(760) 431-7695 or (800) 654-5126
(760) 431-6948 (fax) or (800) 650-5115 (fax)
www.hayhouse.com® • www.hayfoundation.org

Published and distributed in Australia by: Hay House Australia Pty.
Ltd., 18/36 Ralph St., Alexandria NSW 2015 • *Phone:* 612-9669-
4299 • *Fax:* 612-9669-4144 • www.hayhouse.com.au

Published and distributed in the United Kingdom by: Hay House UK,
Ltd., Astley House, 33 Notting Hill Gate, London W11 3JQ • *Phone:*
44-20-3675-2450 • *Fax:* 44-20-3675-2451 • www.hayhouse.co.uk

Published and distributed in the Republic of South Africa by: Hay
House SA (Pty), Ltd., P.O. Box 990, Witkoppen 2068 • *Phone/Fax:*
27-11-467-8904 • www.hayhouse.co.za

Published in India by: Hay House Publishers India, Muskaan
Complex, Plot No. 3, B-2, Vasant Kunj, New Delhi 110 070 • *Phone:*
91-11-4176-1620 • *Fax:* 91-11-4176-1630 • www.hayhouse.co.in

Distributed in Canada by: Raincoast Books, 2440 Viking Way,
Richmond, B.C. V6V 1N2 • *Phone:* 1-800-663-5714
Fax: 1-800-565-3770 • www.raincoast.com

Take Your Soul on a Vacation

Visit www.HealYourLife.com® to regroup, recharge, and reconnect
with your own magnificence. Featuring blogs, mind-body-spirit
news, and life-changing wisdom from Louise Hay and friends.

Visit www.HealYourLife.com today!

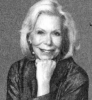
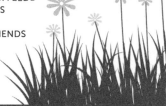